Dietary Fibre and
Related Substances

FOOD SAFETY SERIES

Already Available
Immunoassays for Food Poisoning
Bacteria and Bacterial Toxins
G. M. Wyatt

Food Intolerance
M. H. Lessof

Forthcoming Titles
The *Staphylococci* and their Toxins
M. Bergdoll

The *Aeromonas* Group as a Foodborne Pathogen
S. Palumbo and F. Busta

Food Preservation
G. Gould

Dietary Fibre and Related Substances

I. T. Johnson and D. A. T. Southgate

AFRC Institute of Food Research, Norwich, UK

Springer-Science+Business Media, B.V.

First edition 1994

© 1994 I.T.Johnson and D.A.T.Southgate
Originally published by Chapman & Hall in 1994.
Softcover reprint of the hardcover 1st edition 1994

Typeset in 12/13pt Garamond 3 by Techset Composition Ltd, UK.

ISBN 978-0-412-48470-4   ISBN 978-1-4899-3308-9 (eBook)
DOI 10.1007/978-1-4899-3308-9

A catalogue record for this book is available from the British Library

Contents

Series Introduction

Consumer safety has become a central issue of the food supply system in most countries. It encompasses a large number of interacting scientific and technological matters, such as agricultural practice, microbiology, chemistry, food technology, processing, handling and packaging. The techniques used in understanding and controlling contaminants and toxicity range from the most sophisticated scientific laboratory methods, through industrial engineering science to simple logical rules implemented in the kitchen.

The problems of food safety, however, spread far beyond those directly occupied in food production. Public interest and concern has become acute in recent years, alerting a wide spectrum of specialists in research, education and public affairs.

This series aims to present timely volumes covering all aspects of the subject. They will be up-to-date, specialist reviews written by acknowledged experts in their fields of research to express each author's own viewpoint. The readership is intended to be wide and international, and the style to be comprehensible to non-specialists, albeit professionals.

The series will be of interest to food scientists and technologists working in industry, universities, polytechnics and government institutes; legislators and regulators concerned with the food supply; and specialists in agriculture, engineering, health care and consumer affairs.

One of the most notable developments of recent years in our views about the effect of diet upon health has been in the field of dietary fibre. But although realization of the beneficial role of fibre has entered the public arena, modifying food manufacturing and retailing practice, and changing clinical procedures, there is less awareness of possible adverse effects that may arise.

The authors of this book are recognized internationally as authorities in the field of dietary fibre, and here they have given a definitive account of the present knowledge of the subject. They have also provided, probably for the first time, a wide-ranging description and discussion of the antinutritional and toxicological aspects of high-fibre diets and the regulatory implications. This will be of particular interest and value to professional health workers and legislators, but the book as a whole will be found by all those concerned with our food supply to encompass the whole topic of high-fibre diets in a comprehensible and highly readable way.

J. Edelman

Preface

Opinions vary as to the precise date at which the dietary fibre hypothesis emerged but it is safe to say that it has been a key nutritional concept for nearly a quarter of a century. For much of that time it has been the subject of intense research. Most previous texts have been prepared from papers written for scientific meetings. Inevitably such books tend to focus on new developments in each separate branch of the subject. In this text however we aim to provide the reader with a short but detailed review of the basic concepts surrounding the dietary fibre hypothesis.

The chemistry of cell walls and the problem of analysis are intimately linked, as are the physiological effects of cell wall polysaccharides and the disease states against which dietary fibre is thought to provide protection. This book attempts to provide an integrated and critical review of these issues, assessing both the benefits and possible disadvantages of increased fibre consumption. In keeping with the theme of this series we have focussed particular attention on the food safety issues that surround the consumption of dietary fibre, and which have often been neglected in previous treatments of the subject.

Acknowledgements

The authors would like to thank the staff of the Photography Department of the Institute of Food Research, Norwich laboratory for help with the preparation of figures, and Ms Catherine Reynolds for reading and commenting on the manuscript.

—1—

An Introduction to the Dietary Fibre Hypothesis

—— 1.1 ——
THE ORIGINS OF THE HYPOTHESIS

Although there are many references in the medical and popular literature since the time of Hippocrates to the benefits of consuming unrefined foods, in its current form the 'dietary fibre hypothesis' stems from the writings and lecturing of two medical men, Mr Denis Burkitt and Dr Hugh Trowell, in the early 1970s (*Burkitt & Trowell, 1975*). These two men had both worked in East Africa for a large part of their professional careers and had been intrigued by the differences in the pattern of diseases they saw compared with the Western communities where they had been trained. Trowell was especially interested in the 'metabolic' diseases, obesity, diabetes and coronary heart disease, whereas Burkitt, as a surgeon, was particularly interested in large bowel diseases and especially large bowel cancer. Both men had been influenced by earlier workers, especially ARP Walker working in Southern Africa, and in the popular writing of Surgeon Commander P Cleave who had developed the concept of the 'saccharine diseases' based on the consumption of excessive refined sugars.

In 1971 a paper was published which postulated that diverticular disease was due to a deficiency of fibre in the diet (*Painter & Burkitt, 1971*). This was followed by papers on large bowel cancer and ischaemic heart disease where Trowell (*1972*) used the term 'dietary fibre', which had been used earlier by Hipsley (*1953*), for the constituents of the plant cell walls in the diet (see review by *Southgate, 1992*).

The 'dietary fibre hypothesis' can be expressed formally as follows:

Diets rich in foods containing plant cell wall material in a relatively natural state are protective against a range of diseases that are prevalent in Western affluent communities, for example, diabetes, coronary heart disease, obesity, gall bladder disease, diverticular disease and large bowel cancer.

In some cases the consumption of diets poor in these plant foods may be causative, diverticular disease for example, but in others it may provide the conditions where other aetiological factors become active. The hypothesis is therefore, strictly speaking, one that refers to the protective effects of a type of diet, i.e. one that is rich in plant foods that contain their original cell wall material. Burkitt and Trowell focussed the attention of the clinical world, medical researchers and the general public on the plant cell wall material for which the name 'dietary fibre' became generally accepted. Nevertheless it should not be forgotten that the protective diets that they identified were different in many other ways from the low-fibre diets eaten in Western communities such as the UK and the USA.

These differences are important because they, together with the specific effects of the dietary fibre, contribute to the protective effects (Table 1.1). There is growing recognition that the amount of dietary fibre present in the diet provides a 'marker' for diets that are protective. Thus the consumption of plant foods, especially fruits and vegetables but also cereal foods, brings a range of non-nutrients into the diet which have important biological activity. In this text we will be focussing on dietary fibre and will draw attention to the more important groups of compounds associated with the dietary fibre in plant foods.

The hypothesis proposed by Burkitt and Trowell has proved

Table 1.1 Characteristics of high-fibre diets

Characteristics	Comments
Bulky	Lower physical density g/ml
Energy density	Lower metabolizable energy per unit weight (kcal/kg) but only when fat intakes are also lower
Starch	Proportion of complex carbohydrates: simple sugars increased
Lower-fat	In the context of diets over the world as a whole, the fat also tends to be primarily from vegetable sources and more polyunsaturated
Protein	Vegetable protein sources are more important than animal ones

extremely productive scientifically and current evidence suggests that such high-fibre diets do seem to be protective. However, much of the physiological research that has been carried out since the early 1970s has tended to show that the mechanisms of action originally proposed were naive (Figs 1.1 and 1.2), primarily because they did not take into account the true nature of the chemical and physical properties of the components of the plant cell wall, but also because the research stimulated by the hypothesis has substantially advanced our knowledge of the effects of diet on the gastrointestinal tract.

—— 1.2 ——
THE DEFINITION OF DIETARY FIBRE

Before one can discuss the quantitative effects of dietary fibre it is necessary to examine the problem of definition because this has been a cause of considerable debate since Trowell reused the concept originally introduced by Hipsley. Trowell was convinced that the plant cell walls in the unrefined foods making up the diet of the rural African were the active principles. He first spoke of 'the skeletal remains of the plant cell wall' before adopting the term 'dietary fibre'. At that time he was unaware of the chemistry of the plant cell wall, but he was conscious that the 'fibre' values that had been measured by the food chemists for more than a century were not meaningful measures of what he envisaged as the active components in the protective diets. Burkitt was also aware that these 'fibre' values did not include the major part of the indigestible fraction of human foodstuffs which he had come to believe was important for large bowel function and health.

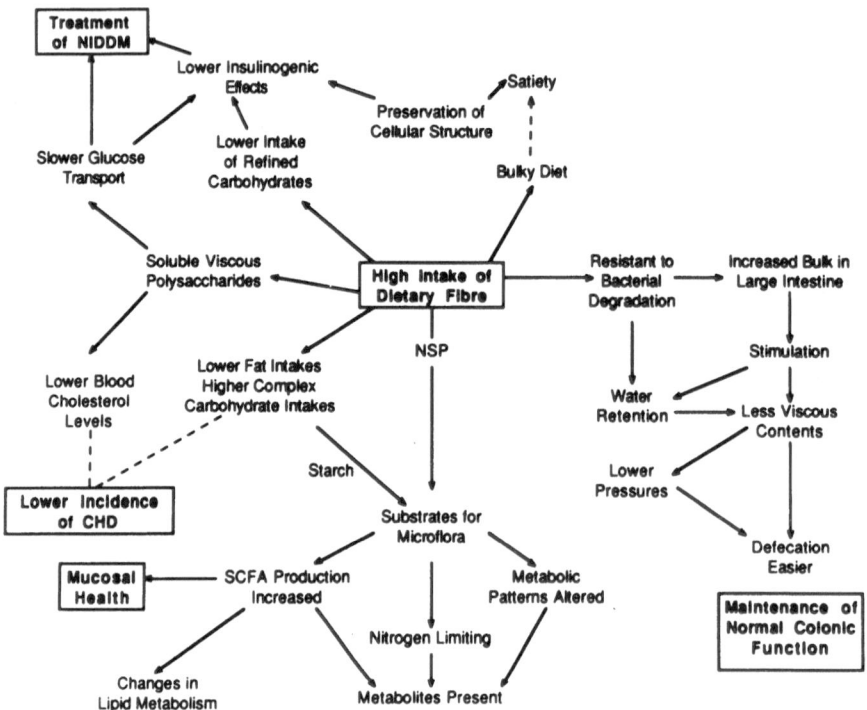

Figure 1.1
Schematic outline of the original hypotheses on the mechanism of action of dietary fibre. (Reproduced from Southgate [1991] *with permission from the* Journal of the Royal Society of Health.)

The use of the word 'fibre' led many researchers to start using the published values for foods. These were 'crude fibre' values which gave a poor measure of the cellulose and lignin in foods, and therefore were insensitive measures of the plant cell wall material in the diet. Other workers turned to the 'detergent fibre' procedures developed by PJ Van Soest (*Van Soest, 1963*), which had been shown to be analytically and conceptually superior to the older crude fibre methods. However, these had been designed for animal feeds and did not measure the soluble components of plant cell walls.

The concept of 'unavailable carbohydrates' originally developed by

Simplified View of Original Concepts

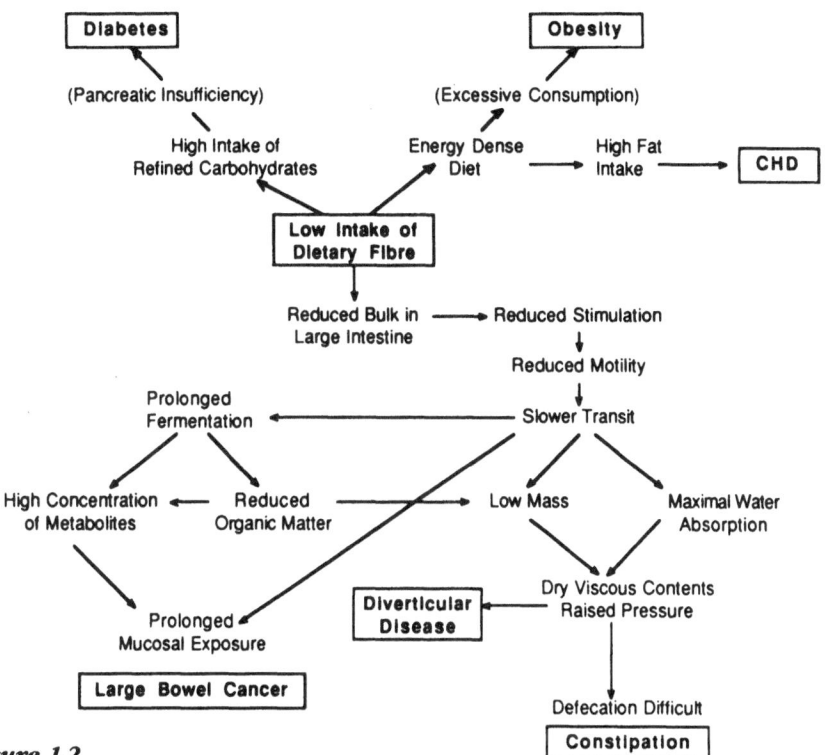

Figure 1.2

Current evidence for the physiological modes of action of dietary fibre. (Reproduced from Southgate [1991] with permission from the Journal of the Royal Society of Health.)

McCance and Lawrence in 1929 included all the constituents of the plant cell wall and in 1976 Trowell and a group of researchers proposed that dietary fibre should be defined as:

> The sum of the lignin and the plant polysaccharides that are not digested by the endogenous secretions of the mammalian digestive tract.

This would include all the major components of the plant cell wall, although it excluded the small amounts of protein, waxes and inorganic material that typically account for less than 10% of the wall. It was recognized that isolated polysaccharides would also be included by this definition. The decision to include such components was deliberate because they were being used, at the time, as 'models' in the study of the physiological effects of dietary fibre, and pragmatic, in that most were structurally related to cell wall constituents and could not be distinguished from them analytically.

—— 1.3 ——
THE ANALYSIS OF DIETARY FIBRE

The establishment of an accepted definition of dietary fibre enabled biomedical researchers and food scientists to use analytical methods developed for unavailable carbohydrates to quantify the dietary fibre in foods, and therefore the diet. This was a major priority for dietary fibre research in the 1970s. Other workers focussed on the indigestibility of dietary fibre and developed 'physiological' methods which incorporated proteolytic and amylolytic enzymatic treatments to remove digestible components, leaving an indigestible dietary fibre residue. The methods used gravimetric assay techniques, and the residue could be used in studies of the properties of isolated dietary fibre preparations (*Asp et al., 1983*). In practice these methods did not differ very greatly from the unavailable carbohydrate procedures, which also employed enzymatic methods to remove starch, but which used colorimetric methods to measure the carbohydrate components directly, followed by the gravimetric measurement of lignin. In practice also, the residue always contained residual protein and it became customary to correct the residue for this. Some starch was subsequently found to be enzymatically resistant and this was included in the gravimetric residue or analysed with the unavailable carbohydrates. This will be discussed in detail later in Chapter 2.

The colorimetric measurement of the carbohydrate constituents in the unavailable carbohydrates developed in the 1960s (*Southgate, 1969*) was prone to mutual interference effects and subsequent developments have used gas-liquid chromatography (GLC) and more recently high-performance liquid chromatography (HPLC). In these methods considerable care has been taken to remove any interference from enzymatically resistant starch and to measure the non-alpha-glucans of the plant cell wall with precision. These methods, which describe the fraction measured unequivocally, have been called the 'non-starch polysaccharide' (NSP) methods (*Englyst & Cummings, 1988*). The fraction measured does not include lignin and is thus formally not identical to dietary fibre as originally defined. However, because the NSP account for about 90% of most plant cell walls their measurement provides a good index of dietary fibre as originally conceived and this method is preferred by the UK Ministry of Agriculture, Fisheries and Food (MAFF) for the nutritional labelling of foods.

The gravimetric indigestible residue procedures have been extensively developed in the USA (*Prosky et al., 1984*) and in some European countries as methods for determining total dietary fibre (TDF), because it is believed that gravimetric methods are simpler, more rapid, require less investment in capital equipment, and are therefore more suitable for regulatory control of labelling.

1.3.1 Differences between the Analytical Methods

The two major types of method in use at the present time give slightly different values for some foods. When making comparisons between the composition of foods or comparing dietary intakes it is important to know the actual method used. In general the gravimetric TDF values are slightly higher than the NSP values, because the former include lignin and resistant starch. The differences are small, and indeed insignificant for most vegetables and fruits, but they may be of the order of 1 g/100 g for unprocessed cereal foods because of the non-inclusion of lignin in NSP values. In heat-processed cereal foods and potato the TDF values may be 2 or 3 g/100 g higher because of the inclusion of resistant starch. The UK tables of food composition 'McCance and Widdowson's The Composition of Food' (*Holland et al., 1991*) give values for two methods: the older, colorimetric 'Southgate' method and the NSP method. The former values are higher because they include lignin and some resistant starch and are similar in magnitude to the TDF values for cereal products.

—— 1.4 ——
INTAKES OF DIETARY FIBRE IN DIFFERENT POPULATIONS

As mentioned above, when making comparisons between estimates of dietary fibre intakes by different populations it is essential to take recognition of the methods used for the dietary fibre values. Much of the comparative data that does exist relates to measurements made using the older 'unavailable carbohydrate' methods, which give higher values than the more recent estimates using NSP techniques. On this basis the distributions of intakes in the UK are skewed. Men have the higher median intake of around 24 g per head per day, with the range between 10 and 45 g. Women have a median intake of about 18 g, with the range between 7.5 and 33 g. In men the intake is not age-related but younger women tend to have higher intakes than older women. The differences between men and women are due, in part, to the different amounts of food eaten by the sexes. However, women in general tend to eat a diet with a higher dietary fibre density than men. Regionally the populations of Scotland and the North of England eat less dietary fibre than those living in Southern counties (*Gregory et al., 1990*). Estimates of NSP intake by the UK population give significantly lower values of between 11 and 13 g per day (*Cummings et al., 1992*). Analyses of trends in consumption of dietary fibre with time show that intakes in the UK have declined over the present century, except for the periods during the 1914–18 and 1939–45 wars when the use of higher-extraction wheat flours in breadmaking and the increased consumption of potatoes resulted in significant increases in dietary fibre intake.

Where data are available, the range of intakes seen in the UK seem to be typical of those for many other developed countries. Intakes tend to be higher in Scandinavian countries where rye and mixtures of wheat and rye flours are used in breadmaking. In the developing countries, intakes tend to be higher because of the greater importance of plant foods and especially cereals. Some African populations may have intakes of up to 100 g per day. In general the average level of fibre in the diet of populations is very dependent on the staple cereal. For example, where rice is the staple intakes are usually comparable to those seen in the UK, but wheat-eaters have considerable higher intakes.

—— 1.5 ——
DIETARY RECOMMENDATIONS FOR THE INTAKE OF DIETARY FIBRE

In the UK and other developed countries the current recommendations for the intake of dietary fibre are based on consideration of the evidence that dietary fibre has specific physiological effects that could be regarded as protective in relation to degenerative diseases. The more important of these diseases and the evidence upon which recommendations are based are briefly summarized below.

1.5.1 Diabetes

There is little evidence to suggest that the low consumption of dietary fibre has a significant effect in the aetiology of non-insulin-dependent diabetes mellitus (NIDDM). This may be primarily because in most epidemiological studies it is not possible to separate the confounding effects of the other attributes of low-fibre diets, for example their high fat content and the higher energy density of such diets when compared with high-fibre diets. There are, however, a substantial number of studies showing improved management of diabetes using high-fibre, low-fat diets. Many viscous polysaccharides improve the glycaemic response to meals in NIDDM, and these polysaccharides are used regularly in the management of the condition. This topic is discussed in detail in Chapter 3.

1.5.2 Obesity

There is growing evidence for an effect of increased intakes of dietary fibre in reducing voluntary food intake because of effects on satiety, but the long-term importance of dietary fibre intake in weight maintenance has yet to be established.

1.5.3 Coronary Heart Disease

Much of the epidemiological evidence linking a high intake of dietary fibre with reduced risk of coronary disease is confounded by the other attributes of high-fibre diets. For example, such diets are often linked with a relatively low fat intake, a potentially beneficial fatty acid ratio and a higher intake of potentially protective vitamins and other substances from the plant foods. However, convincing evidence of a protective relationship has been observed in some studies, and the beneficial effects of high fibre intakes in slowing glucose absorption and effects on insulin secretion may be indicative of a protective action.

1.5.4 Large Bowel Disease

One of the most consistent and widely observed effects of a relatively high dietary fibre intake is increased faecal weight and reduced constipation. This effect, for which the mechanisms are considered in more detail in Chapter 3, is one of the few cases where there is enough information on dose–response relationships to propose quantitative recommendations for intake. International comparisons of NSP intake and faecal weights, and between faecal weights and large bowel cancer rates, show highly significant relationships. These studies show that large bowel cancer rates are highest when stool weights are below 150 g per day. On the basis of a typical UK stool weight of 100 g per day, associated with an NSP intake of between 11 and 13 g per day, it is recommended that the average population intake should rise to 18 g per day with the range from 12 to 24 g (*Department of Health, 1991*). It should be noted that these figures are virtually equivalent to the frequently quoted 30 g per head per day recommended on the basis of the 'Southgate' values in the Nutrition Advisory Committee on Nutrition Education (NACNE) proposal. The current guidelines do not include recommendations for children because no quantitative information upon which to base such recommendations was available to the panel. The evidence that is available suggests that for children a body weight basis for the expression of fibre intake is preferable to an energy intake basis.

The UK recommendation for an increase in NSP intake of around 50% of current levels is similar to the current recommendations in many other countries including the USA and Canada. In Scandinavia the recommendation is couched in nutrient density terms and recommends an intake of 10 g per 10 MJ; this gives figures comparable to the UK recommendations for most of the population, but it does result in high recommended intakes for very active people.

—— 1.6 ——
DIETARY FIBRE, STARCH AND RESISTANT STARCH

Starch and dietary fibre constitute the major types of polysaccharides found in plant foods. In most foods starch is present to a much higher concentration, with starch:dietary fibre ratios as high as 80:1 in some cereal foods. In the classical nutritional textbooks starch was included in the 'available' carbohydrates that were digested and absorbed in the small intestine as glucose. During the development of the NSP methods it became apparent that some starch was resistant to enzymatic hydrolysis under the conditions used. This 'resistant starch' therefore passed into the dietary fibre fraction and elevated it. The resistance of some starch to *in vitro* enzymatic hydrolysis had been recognized for many years by food analysts using treatment with alkali or dimethyl sulphoxide (DMSO) before enzymatic hydrolysis of starch, to disrupt the hydrogen bonding that was believed to be involved. During the course of *in vivo* studies with human subjects it has subsequently become clear that some physiologically resistant starch is invariably present in the material entering the large intestine.

The presence of a resistant starch fraction in foods has attracted a great deal of attention. The first reason for this is that the presence of resistant starch in *in vitro* assays distorts the dietary fibre data. This is important because the resistance is profoundly affected by processing. Foods that are heated in a moist environment and then cooled contain more resistant starch due to the retrogradation of amylose in the food. The second issue is the possible physiological effects of the starch entering the large intestine, and the third is the other physiological or metabolic effects of starch that is absorbed more slowly as short-chain fatty acids from fermentation in the large intestine. Most resistant starch is fermented on reaching the large bowel, although the rate of fermentation varies between forms. The major short-chain fatty acid from this fermentation appears to be butyric acid.

It is now clear that the physiological resistance of starch can be due to a combination of factors that relate to the physical state of the starch in the food. First, some foods have starch granules containing crystalline forms that make them highly resistant to intestinal hydrolysis. These include the starch in unripe bananas and in raw potatoes. Second, the starch granules may be physically trapped within the plant–food matrix so that the granules cannot swell and are therefore protected physically. Third, the amylose moiety of the starch molecules can undergo 'retrogradation' and form, by hydrogen bonding, an insoluble and highly resistant semicrystalline structure. Changes in the susceptibility to digestive enzymes of purified pea-amylose, after gelatinization and different periods of cooling, are illustrated in Fig. 1.3. Similar effects occur in whole peas that have been cooked normally and then stored at a low temperature. Physiologically resistant starch results from a combination of the three effects. However, from an analytical point of view, retrograded amylose is the major resistant starch component in the TDF residues, and in the NSP residues if the samples have not been treated with DMSO.

Apart from these effects, the physical treatment of starchy foods

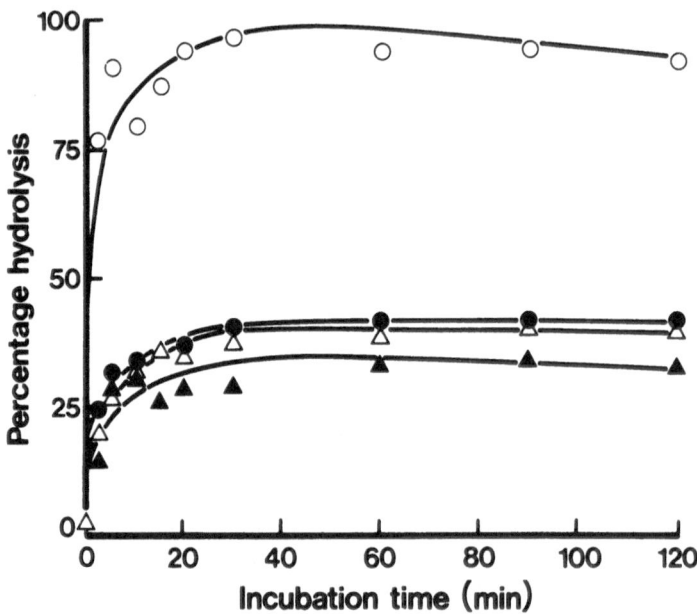

Figure 1.3
Time course for the in vitro *hydrolysis of amylose extracted and purified from peas. The starch was hydrolysed immediately after gelatinization (O), after storage for 1 hour (●) or 4 hours (△) at 20°C, or for 18 hours (▲) at 5°C. (Reproduced from Ring et al. [1988] with permission from Elsevier Applied Science Publishers Ltd.)*

during processing can slow the rate of starch digestion; thus pasta-making produces a slowly hydrolysed starch. Many seed legumes have slowly hydrolysable starch, which is probably due to the presence of cell walls slowing either the swelling of the starch granule or the diffusion of enzymes and the products of digestion. This particular property of cell walls will be discussed in more detail in Chapter 2.

FURTHER READING

British Nutrition Foundation. *Complex Carbohydrates in Foods. Report of the British Nutrition Foundation Task Force.* London: Chapman and Hall, 1991.
Burkitt DP, Trowell HC, eds. *Refined Carbohydrate Foods: Some Implications of Dietary Fibre.* London: Academic Press, 1975.

Schweizer TF, Edwards CA, eds. *Dietary Fibre: A Component of Food*. London: Springer Verlag, 1992.

Southgate DAT. Dietary fibre and the diseases of affluence. In: *A Balanced Diet?* Dobbing J, ed. London: Springer Verlag, 1988, pp 117–39.

Southgate DAT. The dietary fibre hypothesis: A historical perspective. In: *Dietary Fibre: A Component of Food*. Schweizer TF, Edwards CA, eds. London: Springer Verlag, 1992, pp 3–20.

Trowell H, Burkitt D, Heaton K, eds. *Dietary Fibre, Fibre-Depleted Foods and Disease*. London: Academic Press, 1985.

CHAPTER

—2—

Sources, Chemical Composition and Analysis of Dietary Fibre

As we have seen, the term 'dietary fibre' was originally used as a shorthand term for the constituents of the plant cell wall. Furthermore, in the case of the protective diets postulated by Burkitt and Trowell, the distinguishing feature that was considered most important was the consumption of plant foods that contained their cell walls in a relatively natural state. These are, principally, high-extraction (unrefined) cereal foods, vegetables and fruits. Conversely, the low-fibre diets were characterized by a high proportion of plant foods that had had their content of cell wall material reduced by processing and refining. This implies that the most appropriate primary definition for 'dietary fibre' is 'the plant cell wall material in foods and the diet'. In discussing the sources and chemistry of dietary fibre, therefore, the starting point must be a consideration of the plant cell walls in foods. When we move to considering the analytical measurement of dietary fibre we have to consider how this primary definition can best be interpreted in practical terms.

——2.1——
PLANT CELL WALLS IN FOODS

The human diet uses foods derived from a wide range of plants. The range of the parts of the plant consumed is also very wide, including for example the leaves and stems, roots and tubers, flowers, fruits and seeds. These different parts of the plant are made up of various types of tissues, each with its own characteristic types of cell walls These confer a second level of variability over and above that due to the differences in the cell walls of different species (Table 2.1). This means that the dietary fibre in any mixed diet, and indeed in most foods, is derived from a range of types of cell wall structures with compositions that vary depending on the species, the plant organ and the amounts of the different plant foods consumed. The corollary of this is that dietary fibre is not a single homogeneous entity. It is invariably a mixture. Only under experimental conditions, where for example an isolated polysaccharide is being fed, can the dietary fibre be regarded as a single substance.

2.1.1 General Features of the Plant Cell Wall.

Despite the wide variation in the physical structure and detailed chemical composition of the plant cell walls from different foods, it is possible to make some generalizations (*Southgate, 1976a; Selvendran, 1984*). The typical cell type making up the flesh of fruits and vegetables is the undifferentiated parenchyma cell. The walls of these cells are typically thin. During the development of the wall the first structure to form is the middle lamella, which is characteristically rich in uronic acid containing polysaccharides (uronans). The primary wall is laid down on this structure

Table 2.1 Heterogeneity of plant foods in the diet and the effects on the composition of plant cell wall material.

Major variable	Examples	Effects on dietary fibre
Types of plant organ consumed	Roots/tubers, stems, petioles, leaves, flowers/flower buds, seeds	Types of polysaccharide present Organization within cell wall architecture
Types of plant cell wall structures consumed	Parenchyma, conducting tissues (phloem, xylem), supporting tissues (collenchyma, sclerenchyma), epidermal tissues	Presence of associated proteins, lignins, cutins, suberins and inorganic materials

15

with the cellulose fibrils forming initially as a random network in a matrix of primarily water-soluble, arabinogalactan polysaccharides. In the secondary wall the cellulose fibrils become orientated in parallel sheets, and the matrix polysaccharides comprise a wider range of polysaccharides, including various branched and substituted xylans. In the primary wall glycoproteins are present at about 10% of the dry wall, and appear to play an important role in the orientation of the polysaccharide structures.

Other cell wall types develop in a similar way initially. The wall may thicken by the formation of additional layers of cellulose and matrix polysaccharides to form the supporting collenchyma tissue. In the vascular bundles of the plant, the deposition of lignin starts in the xylem vessels. In the early stages this aromatic polymer, which is formed by the condensation of phenolic alcohols, develops as annular regions or as spirals within the matrix of the wall. In some tissues the lignification becomes very extensive as they mature, and in woody tissues extends throughout the wall matrix forming dead conducting or supporting structures. In leaves and stems the outer epidermal tissues of the plant frequently have complex lipids on their external surfaces. These cutins are internal esters of long-chain hydroxy aliphatic acids and are virtually integral parts of these external walls. In the external tissues of roots and tubers and some fruits, an analogous substance suberin is formed. Both these lipids and the lignin create hydrophobic regions in the walls.

The tissues of fruits frequently contain special types of cell walls. The outer layers may develop thickened walls where lignin and the complex polyphenolic substances, the tannins, are deposited. These give the wall structural rigidity and protect the fruit and seeds from desiccation and predation. In other fruits, cells rich in water-soluble mucilages may be formed.

Seed structures within the fruits typically have tough lignified seed coats, again as protective structures against desiccation. Within the seed the structures are very dependent on the species. In seed legumes there may be large cotyledons, which consist of undifferentiated cells, usually containing lipid or starch as the food source for germination; other species have endospermal tissues similarly rich in storage lipids or polysaccharides. The embryo is made up of thin-walled, partially differentiated stem and root structures. In cereal grains the outer layers are usually thick-walled and rich in lignin and polyphenolic materials. The embryo or germ is a small part of the seed with thin-walled, partially differentiated tissues, and the bulk of the seed is made up of thin-walled endospermal cells filled with starch granules.

2.1.2 Composition of the Plant Cell Wall

The types of polysaccharide present are characteristic of the plant and tissue but, as with structural features, it is possible to make some generalizations. In the immature, undifferentiated wall about 75–80% of the dry wall is polysaccharide in nature with about 10% of protein and about 4% of lipid constituents. Cellulose makes up about one-third of the total polysaccharide and the remainder is non-cellulosic polysaccharide (Table 2.2). In the classical analytical fractionations of the plant cell wall it was customary to divide the wall into three fractions depending on solubility in water and different strengths of alkali. These fractions are: pectic substances, soluble in water (usually hot with a chelating agent); hemicelluloses, insoluble in water but soluble in dilute alkali; and alpha-cellulose, insoluble in strong alkali. The fractions obtained were to a considerable extent artefacts of the fractionation and did not necessarily correspond to chemically defined groups of substances (*Albersheim, 1965*). For this reason many workers in the field think that it is better to talk of two polysaccharide fractions: a cellulose, or possibly cellulosic polysaccharide fraction; and the non-cellulosic polysaccharides (NCP). This latter group includes a spectrum of polysaccharides ranging from those rich in uronic acids (uronans, the major components of pectin) to those containing low concentrations of uronic acids, the neutral polysaccharides which contain arabinose, galactose, mannose, xylose and glucose as constituent monomers. (See Table 2.3.)

Table 2.2 Typical values for overall composition of plant cell wall material

	Runner bean pods				Wheat bran
Constituent	Primary wall		Secondary wall		Mature wall
	Fresh basis	Dry basis	Fresh basis	Dry basis	Dry basis
Water	70	—	15	—	—
Cellulose	10	33.2	35	41	18.9
Pectic substances	12	40.0	25	6	2.0
Hemicellulose	6	20.0	25	29	53.5
Glycoprotein	2	7.0	2	2	—
Lignin	0	0	18	21	12.1

Table 2.3 Polysaccharides in plant materials

Primary source	Major groups	Components present
Structural materials of the plant cell wall	Cellulose, non-cellulosic polysaccharides	Pectic substances, hemi-celluloses
Non-structural polysaccharides	Gums, mucilages	
Polysaccharide food additives	Gums, algal polysaccharides, modified celluloses, modified starches	Guar, locust bean, alginates, carrageenan
Associated substances	Lignin, cutin, suberin	

When the wall matures the proportion of carbohydrate increases as the wall expands in volume, so that the concentration of protein declines to around 3–4%; at the same time the process of lignification adds lignin to the wall. Lignin forms within the matrix, infiltrating and forming covalent links with the carbohydrates. This leads to an increase in the volume of the wall, in which lignin may account for about 17%, leaving the carbohydrates to make up about 80%. In only partially lignified walls the polysaccharide content approaches 90%.

In the immature wall the NCP of the matrix are mainly water-soluble, consisting of arabinogalactans and galacturonorhamnans (polymers of galacturonic acid with rhamnose insertions in the chain). As the wall matures, other NCP are formed comprising glucoxylans, and a range of substituted xylans with arabinosyl and methylglucuronosyl side chains. In general the more highly branched and substituted polymers are water-soluble and the more linear ones insoluble. In the cell walls of fruits and vegetables the arabinogalactans are the characteristic NCP. In cereal foods, insoluble arabinoxylans are the major NCP of wheat and rye, while oats and barley contain, in addition, branched beta-glucans which are soluble in water.

2.1.3 Macromolecular Character of the Cell Wall

The polysaccharide components of the cell wall are arranged in ordered structures which confer a macromolecular organisation on the wall. Thus the cellulose molecules are organized into cellulose fibrils which are covered with a sheath of glucoxylan. The galacturonorhamnans are linked to arabinogalactans which appear to be covalently attached to the protein via the arabinosyl chains. In the living plant this matrix is normally fully hydrated. In the immature wall the water content may be as high as 70%

but this falls as the wall matures and as the three-dimensional molecules of lignin infiltrate the matrix, creating hydrophobic regions. It is important, when considering the properties of dietary fibre in a diet, to take account of the structural organization within the wall, the type of cell wall within the plant tissues and also the nature of the tissues in the plant foods consumed. Each of these levels of structural organization modifies the physical and chemical properties of the dietary fibre.

——2.2——
CHEMISTRY OF THE POLYSACCHARIDES

The polysaccharides of the plant cell walls in foods make up the major components of dietary fibre and are responsible for the majority of the physiological effects of dietary fibre. However, the aromatic polymer lignin, because of its intimate association within the cell wall matrix, has important effects in modifying the properties of the polysaccharides.

In processed foods a wide range of polysaccharides are used as additives, principally to modify or control the physical properties of the product. Many of these polysaccharides are derived from cell wall structures and share the chemical structural features of the plant cell wall components. Since these polysaccharides cannot be distinguished analytically from analogous components in the walls it is necessary to discuss them in this section on the chemistry of the polysaccharides of dietary fibre. The major common feature of these polysaccharides lies in the glycosidic bonds they contain. Unlike the major plant polysaccharide starch, they do not contain alpha-glucosidic bonds; they are non-alpha-glucans or non-starch polysaccharides. (This is a trivial name which is not strictly correct since the alpha-glucans include glycogen, found in some fungi, and laminarin, a polysaccharide in the alga Laminaria.)

——2.3——
CLASSIFICATION OF THE NON-STARCH POLYSACCHARIDES IN FOODS

It is possible to classify the NSP in many different ways but one of the most useful as a starting point is to examine them according to their role in the plant and then to consider how this can be interpreted physiologi-cally (Table 2.4).

2.3.1 Structural Materials of the Plant Cell Wall

For the reasons given earlier the polysaccharides fall into two major categories, cellulosic and non-cellulosic.

Cellulosic polysaccharides

The major polysaccharide of this group is cellulose, which is a linear beta-linked glucan of high molecular weight, ranging between 500,000 and 1 million Daltons. The polydisperse nature of isolated cellulose may be an artefact of the extraction conditions used because many methods involve the use of vigorous oxidizing conditions to remove the lignin associated with the cellulose. The conformation imposed by the beta linkages facilitates hydrogen bonding between parallel chains, leading to the characteristic cellulose fibrils and the macroscopic cellulose fibres found for example in cotton. This bonding confers crystalline properties on the cellulose.

Cellulose is rather inert; it will absorb modest amounts of water but chemical reactions only occur if the material has been swollen in acid or solvents which disrupt the hydrogen bonding. Oxidation of the end groups can occur during isolation and these together with dis-ordered regions of the molecule act as the initiating areas for sub-stitution reactions. One should therefore be cautious when interpreting the effects of an isolated cellulose as characteristic of a general effect of all celluloses.

Cellulose fibres can adsorb small molecules on their surfaces because the external hydroxyl groups have weak acidic properties and can also hydrogen bond. Prolonged milling in a ball-mill can depolymerize the cellulose molecules, leading to greatly reduced chain lengths; these preparations, sometimes called alpha-cellulose, can be made water-dispersible and are used as bulking agents in foods.

Non-cellulosic polysaccharides

This category includes a very wide variety of types of polysaccharide. Most contain at least two, and usually more, monosaccharide or uronic acid components, but in general they have backbone structures of one monosaccharide.

Table 2.4 Classification of plant polysaccharides

Role in the plant/food	Types of polysaccharides	Analytical classification	Site of digestion	Products of digestion	Physiological classification
Storage polysaccharides	Starch: amylose, amylopectin Fructans Galactomannans	Alpha-glucans Non-alpha-glucans	Small intestine (enzymatic)	Mono- and di-saccharides	Available carbohydrates
Structural components of the plant cell walls	Non-cellulosic: pectins, hemi-cellulose, Cellulose	Non-starch poly-saccharides	Large intestine (microbial)	Short-chain fatty acids: acetate, proprionate, butyrate	Unavailable carbohydrates
Isolated polysaccharides occurring naturally	Gums, mucilages			Carbon dioxide, hydrogen, methane	
Polysaccharide food additives	Pectin, Gums, algal polysaccharides, modified cell-ulose, Modified starches				

Uronic acid polymers

The major uronan in land plants is a polymer of galacturonic acid which has rhamnose insertions at intervals. Pectin is often seen as the typical molecule, but in practice most pectins have been depolymerized during extraction, and arabinosyl and galactosyl residues are probably present on the native molecule in the wall. The carboxyl groups are esterified with methyl alcohol to a variable extent in different plants; citrus plants, for example, are usually highly methoxylated whereas the strawberry is a low methoxy plant. In many plants the groups are acetylated. Carboxyl groups that are not esterified are capable of forming salts with cations, and divalent cations such as calcium are strongly chelated by these molecules. This is the reason why chelating agents such as ammonium oxalate or EDTA are used in the extraction of these components. The uronans are water-soluble and form the major part of the 'pectic substances' in classical fractionations.

Galactose polymers

The major polymers with galactose backbones are arabinogalactans which form the other main component of the water-soluble 'pectic substances' fraction. The main chain is beta 1–4 linked, with arabinosyl residues on some of the galactose units. Galactans without these side chains have been reported from some food plants such as the potato.

Arabinose polymers

Arabinans have also been isolated from some immature leaves; they are in general highly branched and water-soluble.

Xylan polymers

A wide range of xylans have been isolated. They constitute the major polysaccharides appearing in the 'hemicellulose' fractions, although some can be extracted with water as well. Xylans with glucuronic acid side chains are found in many vegetables. In cereals these may also have arabinose side chains, and there are a wide range of arabinoxylans, some of which are very highly branched.

Branched and substituted glucose polymers

Cellulose is virtually a linear pure glucan and a range of branched and substituted beta-linked glucans of lower molecular weight are found in plant cell walls. Virtually all primary walls contain xyloglucans where up to half the glucose residues carry xylose side chains, often with other sugars such as galactose, fucose and arabinose being present. Cereals also contain mixed linkage beta-glucans with beta 1–3 and 1–4 glucose linked residues in their endospermal walls. The concentrations of these beta-glucans are higher in oats and barley where they make up the major part of the water-soluble fraction.

Mannose polymers

Mannans are found in many plant cell walls, especially in those legumes that have endospermic seeds. Strictly speaking, they are storage polysaccharides, having an analogous role to starch in other seeds. They are, however, stored in the wall, and therefore need to be mentioned here. The beta 1–4 mannan backbone is conformationally very similar to that of cellulose, and pure mannans are extremely insoluble and tough materials and can be worked like wood. In some legumes the chain carries branches of single galactose residues. This radically changes the physical properties to give water-soluble polysaccharides that form viscous solutions and associate with other polysaccharides to form gels. These galactomannans include guar, locust bean and carob bean gums that are widely used as food additives (thickening agents).

2.3.2   Non-Structural Non-Starch Polysaccharides

In addition to the structural polysaccharides, many plant foods contain NSP that are not present in the walls; these include soluble galacturonans found in cell sap, and a range of gums and mucilages. The gums, of which the exudate gums are the best known, are formed in response to physical damage of the plant and serve to restrict water loss; the mucilages are most frequently associated with fruits and seeds, where they act to retain water. These polymers are usually complex, highly branched heteropolysaccharides containing a wide range of monosaccharide and uronic acid residues.

2.3.3   Polysaccharide Food Additives

These form an additional group of NSP found in many processed foods. The amounts present in particular foods vary but the concentrations used are usually low (of the order of 0.5–2%). These polysaccharides are minor constituents of the diet which collectively contribute only around a few hundred milligrams a day to the diet as a whole. Many have been used as 'models' for the polysaccharide components of the plant cell wall, and their physiological effects have been studied largely at what must be regarded as 'pharmacological dose' levels rather than as constituents of the diet. Many are derived from plant cell wall material of land plants but there is an important group derived from the extraction of marine algae (Table 2.4).

Modified celluloses

Esterification and etherification of the hydroxyl groups is used to produce a range of modified celluloses. The methyl- and carboxymethylcelluloses form viscous solutions in water and have been used as thickening agents. The properties of the molecule can be controlled by limiting the extent of substitution and a wide range of different commercial products are available.

Modified pectins

Pectin has long been used to impart a high viscosity to jams and other traditional fruit preserves. The commercial ingredient is prepared by acid extraction of citrus or apple residues and is extensively depolymerized in the process so that the galacturonorhamnan backbone has had most of the side chains removed. The extent of methoxylation determines the gelling capacity in acid sugar solutions, and hence the value of the pectin in jam-making. Amidated pectins are used where more stable polymers are required.

Storage polysaccharides

The use of galactomannans has been mentioned earlier. Guar and locust bean gums are widely used as thickening agents in many processed foods. In guar gum, one in two of the mannose residues in the backbone has a galactose side chain, whereas in locust bean gum about one in four or five has a galactose residue.

2.3.4 Algal Polysaccharides

Alginates

These are widely used in many foods from ice creams to beers. The alginates are copolymers of guluronic and mannuronic acids and can be used as their salts or the free acidic polymer. They are widely used to control foams and can be used in conjunction with divalent ions such as calcium to produce gels of varying stiffness. The properties depend on the ratio of the two uronic acids and lengths of the blocks of them in the chain. A wide range of alginates are available commercially.

Carrageenans

A range of different carrageenans are known, and these are designated by Greek characters. The polymers are unusual in that they contain desoxy sugars and also have sulphated galactose residues. They are acidic polymers and act synergistically with proteins and other polysaccharides to produce a range of gels and viscosities. Because of concerns about the possibly hazardous biological effects of depolymerized acidic fragments, their use is controlled very strictly and only high molecular weight forms are used.

Agar

This is a mixed polysaccharide also containing desoxygalactose sulphate esters and glucuronic acid. The neutral agarose component has the better gelling properties.

2.3.5 Fermentation Gums

Many bacteria produce extracellular polysaccharides which diffuse into the fermentation media. Some of these have interesting physical properties and one, xanthan gum from *Xanthomonas campestris*, has met the required toxicological standards and is permitted in foods. It may be anticipated that more gums from this origin will eventually be approved. It is a beta-glucan with alternating residues, having a two mannose and one glucuronic side chain, some of which terminate in a pyruvate residue; the polymer acts synergistically with some galactomannans.

——2.4——
ANALYTICAL MEASUREMENT OF DIETARY FIBRE

As will be evident from the description of the range of polysaccharides present in the plant cell wall, and the other chemically related polysaccharides found in foods, the problems posed to the analyst in the design of methods for measuring dietary fibre are very considerable. Intuitively one might suppose that the ideal method would involve the fractionation and measurement of all the polysaccharide species present. Such an approach would demand a method specifically designed for each food or mixed diet, and it would also entail a monumental task to complete such an analysis for each food. It is necessary therefore to accept some compromise in order to devise an analytical scheme that will serve the purposes for which the analysis is being undertaken. In many respects the debate that has taken place during the 1980s on the most appropriate method of fibre analysis reflects a lack of recognition that every analytical method has to be considered in the context for which it is designed. Thus the needs of a researcher studying the physiological properties of dietary fibre demand a method that will serve to predict the physiological effects. Likewise the epidemiologist requires a characterization of the dietary fibre intake that can be linked to possible aetiological mechanisms. For regulatory purposes a robust, reproducible and rapid method using, if possible, simple apparatus and unskilled technicians is the ideal. These two approaches may not be mutually exclusive with a relatively simple analyte, but this is not the case with dietary fibre. In practice compromise is inevitable but one must work to ensure that the different types of method are comparable and give similar results.

2.4.1 Measurement of Plant Cell Wall Material

The techniques developed for the study of the plant cell wall provide the most complete and comprehensive methods, and these should form the primary reference point for consideration of the analysis of dietary fibre. They involve detailed sequential extraction under closely controlled conditions, followed by isolation and further fractionation, usually using chromatographic means, then characterization of the component monosaccharides and structural analysis by methylation and mass spectrometry. The rigorous conditions of the classical fractionations with water and alkali have been modified by the introduction of milder conditions and the use of reducing agents to prevent oxidative modification. All the extractions are carried out under closely controlled conditions of temperature and pH. Such methods are very time-consuming, and therefore impracticable for most of the purposes for which dietary fibre analyses are carried out. They should be regarded however as the ultimate reference method, and the review by Selvendran and O'Neill (*1987*) gives a good account of the attention to detail that is required in these types of analysis.

It is possible to divide the major approaches into three main categories (*Southgate, 1976a,b*). These are: a) the methods derived from the classical fibre methods; b) those that start from the concept of indigestible residues in foods; and c) those based on the nutritional classification of the carbohydrates into 'available' and 'unavailable' groups. This order is to a large extent chronological and the methods will be described in this sequence.

2.4.2 Methods Derived from the Classical Fibre Concept

The crude fibre method, developed in the 1860s for the analysis of cattle feeds, is technically exacting but unsuitable in the context of human nutrition. Many authors have shown that it is an unreliable predictor of the indigestible component of animal feeds. Much effort has been made to resolve the technical problems but the major advance was made by PJ Van Soest, who developed a series of methods based on the use of detergents in the extracting solutions. These served to reduce nitrogenous contamination of the residues, and assisted in the effective extraction of forages. The first method, 'acid-detergent fibre' (ADF), involved treatment with Normal (0.5 M) sulphuric acid. This gave a residue that included virtually all the cellulose and lignin in a feed. This residue also contained cutin, suberin and silica and methods were devised for these components, starting with the ADF residue. The second method, 'neutral detergent fibre' (NDF), involved extraction with hot detergent; this left a residue of the insoluble components of the plant cell walls in the feed. All the series of methods are described with practical details in Goering and Van Soest (*1970*). When these methods were applied to human foods there were found to be two problems. First, the soluble components were lost in the NDF extract and could only be recovered from this extract with difficulty. Second, when starch-rich foods were analysed some starch was retained in the NDF residue, resulting in an overestimation of the plant cell wall components. Techniques were evolved to treat the residue with amylase to remove the residual starch but the loss of insoluble components represents a fatal problem, and therefore the method has limited application.

2.4.3 Methods for Indigestible Residue

The earliest method of this type was proposed by Williams and Olmsted in the 1930s as a replacement for crude fibre that was conceptually closer to the indigestible material in human foods and diets. In principle the food was treated with pepsin and pancreatin, to remove the protein and starch respectively, and the residue was hydrolysed sequentially in two strengths of sulphuric acid. The carbohydrates were measured as reducing sugars in the hydrolysates, with the residual lignin being measured gravimetrically. Hellendoorn et al. (*1975*) proposed a very similar approach, arguing that the residue was a better way of measuring dietary fibre. The residue was measured gravimetrically and the residual protein and starch were regarded by the author as being measures of the indigestibility of these components. It was argued therefore that they should properly be included in 'dietary fibre' estimates. This approach was regarded as a 'physiological' one because it used enzymes to extract the other components of foods, and the residue itself, which had not been vigorously treated, was seen as providing a dietary fibre preparation that could be used for studies of the binding of water and cations and for measuring fermentability in *in vitro* systems. The method was developed in Sweden by Asp (*Asp et al., 1983*) and later in Switzerland by Schweizer (*1989*), and was used to form the basis for the Association of Official Analytic Chemists (AOAC) method of Prosky et al. (*1984; 1988*).

The principles of the method are illustrated schematically in Fig. 2.1.

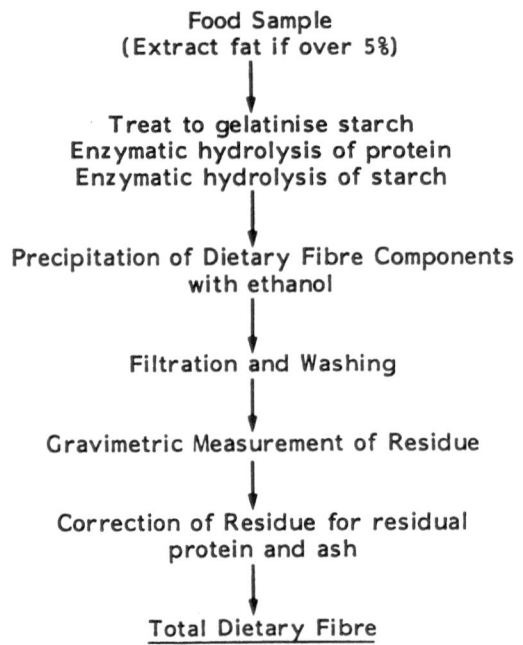

Food Sample
(Extract fat if over 5%)

↓

Treat to gelatinise starch
Enzymatic hydrolysis of protein
Enzymatic hydrolysis of starch

↓

Precipitation of Dietary Fibre Components
with ethanol

↓

Filtration and Washing

↓

Gravimetric Measurement of Residue

↓

Correction of Residue for residual
protein and ash

↓

Total Dietary Fibre

Figure 2.1

Schematic flow chart for the measurement of total dietary fibre by the AOAC method.

The food is treated with pepsin, and then with two amylase preparations, a thermally stable one first, and then amyloglucosidase. The hydrolysate is treated with alcohol to precipitate the dietary fibre residue which is filtered off, washed and weighed. The residue weight is corrected for protein by measuring total nitrogen and calculating the crude protein content (N × 6.25); the residual ash is measured. These are deducted from the residue weight to give a total dietary fibre (TDF) value. If the monosaccharide content is required the residue can be hydrolysed and the sugars measured by GLC or HPLC.

This method has been subjected to collaborative trials and its performance is judged satisfactory for acceptance as an Official Method by the AOAC. The method has some technical limitations when used for measuring low concentrations of TDF because the sample size is limited. This means that the gravimetric approach requires high precision in the measurement of blanks and the corrections for protein and ash. Some residues are difficult to filter quickly and these tend to be most affected by co-precipitation effects. Heat-induced artefacts from proteins cause interference and the values include some enzymatically resistant starch in addition to NSP and lignin. As a general rule the TDF values tend to overestimate the plant cell wall materials in foods but this is most significant at the lower end of the concentration range.

2.4.4 Methods for Unavailable Carbohydrates

McCance and Lawrence (1929) proposed that for nutritional purposes the food carbohydrates could be considered to fall into two groups. These comprised the 'available carbohydrates', which included the free sugars and starch that were digested and absorbed as carbohydrate in the small intestine, and the 'unavailable carbohydrates', which were not digested by the intestinal secretions and therefore did not yield carbohydrates for absorption. The latter do however provide short-chain fatty acids from fermentation in the large intestine. In this original terminology the 'unavailable' term referred to the carbohydrate, not to energy as some recent workers have implied. Methods were derived in the 1930s to measure this fraction by deducting the protein and starch values (obtained after amylolytic hydrolysis using a fungal enzyme preparation) from the residue of the food insoluble in 80% v/v ethanol. These values were published in the 1st, 2nd and 3rd editions of *The Composition of Foods* (McCance & Widdowson, 1940; 1946; 1960).

This approach was developed further by Southgate when designing methods for these carbohydrates in the period 1959–69 (*Southgate, 1969*), using sequential hydrolysis and specific colorimetric methods for the major classes of components of plant cell walls (pentose, hexoses and uronic acids), and gravimetric analysis of Klason lignin. These measurements formed the basis for the values published in 1978 in the 4th edition of *The Composition of Foods* (*Paul & Southgate, 1978*). Because they constituted the first attempt to provide a systematic coverage of foods, these values have since been widely used.

Early in 1976 it became clear that GLC now provided a more specific way for measuring the component sugars and, after some early collaboration, HN Englyst began to develop these more detailed methods. Early on it was realized that some enzymatically resistant starch was present in the unavailable carbohydrate fraction, and techniques were introduced to remove this so that reliable values for the plant cell wall NSP could be obtained (*Englyst et al., 1982*). The sample size for these methods precluded the measurement of lignin but it was considered better to measure this cell wall component separately because of its own specific properties. The amounts of lignin in most foods are low so no major underestimation was produced. The method is illustrated schematically in

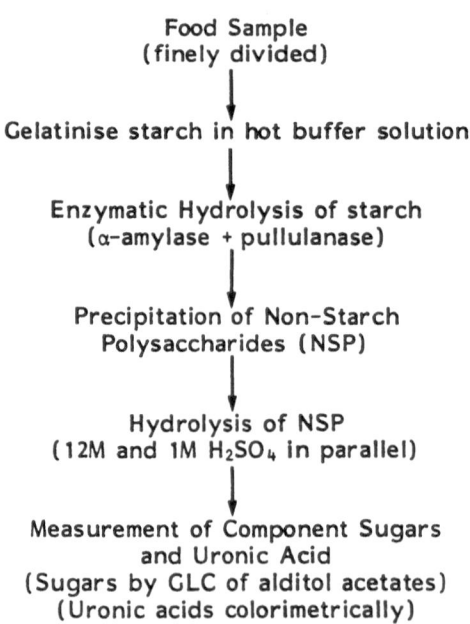

Food Sample
(finely divided)

↓

Gelatinise starch in hot buffer solution

↓

Enzymatic Hydrolysis of starch
(α-amylase + pullulanase)

↓

Precipitation of Non-Starch
Polysaccharides (NSP)

↓

Hydrolysis of NSP
(12M and 1M H_2SO_4 in parallel)

↓

Measurement of Component Sugars
and Uronic Acid
(Sugars by GLC of alditol acetates)
(Uronic acids colorimetrically)

Figure 2.2
Schematic flow chart for the measurement of non-starch polysaccharides by the englyst method.

Fig. 2.2. The sample is treated with DMSO to solubilize resistant starch and then with a thermally stable amylase to gelatinize the starch. Amylase and pullulanase are then added to complete the starch hydrolysis and the unhydrolysed NSP are precipitated with ethanol at 80% by volume. The residue is dried and dispersed in 12 M sulphuric acid, which is later diluted and heated to complete the hydrolysis of the polysaccharides. The monosaccharides are reduced to their alditols and derivatized and measured as the alditol acetates by GLC. They can also be measured directly by HPLC or as a total value colorimetrically. The method has gone through a large number of modifications to improve technical features and these methods have also been the subject of several collaborative trials. The precision of the method can be a problem in inexperienced hands, especially when sampling heterogeneous foods, using a small initial sample size (50–200 mg). In general, because they do not measure lignin, the NSP methods tend to underestimate plant cell wall material slightly; the underestimation is most pronounced at the higher concentrations because these are typically cereal foods with up to 2 g/100 g of lignin (Fig. 2.3).

2.4.5 Comparison of Different Methodological Approaches

During the early 1990s the TDF method of the AOAC and the NSP method of Englyst have become the major contenders for adoption as the preferred method for measuring dietary fibre for food labelling purposes. The proponents of the two methods and the debates that have ensued have tended to emphasize the differences between the methods and to elevate them to differences of principle. If one considers the diagram (Fig. 2.4.) one can see how the different approaches to measuring and classifying the polysaccharides are related to one another. In a major review of analytical methodology, Asp et al. (1992) showed how the methods have evolved, and emphasized the similarities. Thus all existing methods use an enzymatic stage to remove starch. The gravimetric measurement of the residue is bypassed in the NSP method, in favour of going directly to the carbohydrates analysis; such an end-point can be reached in the AOAC TDF method but only after the residue has been weighed. In the development of the Southgate method the gravimetric assay was available, but it was never considered to be a viable option because of the technical difficulties of collecting and weighing the small residues from some foods. Coupled with this was a conceptual prejudice

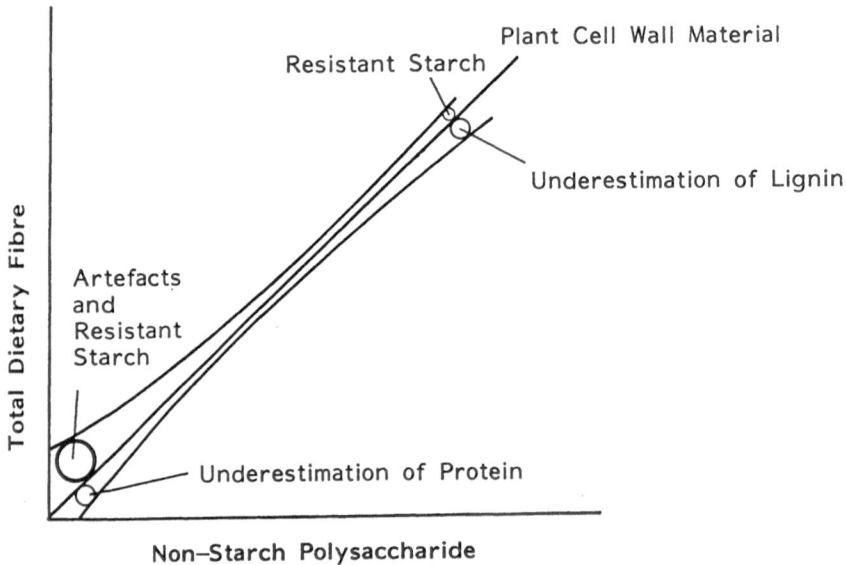

Figure 2.3

The diagram shows the theoretical relationship between the total dietary fibre (TDF) values, non-starch polysaccharide (NSP) values and plant cell wall material (PCWM), which is represented by the central line on the figure. TDF values tend to overestimate PCWM at all levels because of the inclusion of resistant starch; the overestimation is increased at low levels of PCWM because of the inclusion of non-carbohydrate artifacts in the gravimetric residue. NSP values tend to underestimate PCWM at all levels because of the exclusion of lignin and cell wall protein. At higher levels the underestimation is primarily due to lignin and at lower levels to cell wall protein.

in favour of direct measurement of the carbohydrates either by colorimetric techniques or, more specifically, by GLC or HPLC. This position is still recommended to the reader as being technically and conceptually preferable to measuring a residue of unknown composition.

As outlined earlier, in Chapter 1, the TDF method gives very similar results to the NSP method for fruits and vegetables. For unprocessed cereals the TDF values are higher because they include lignin and with processed cereals most TDF values are higher because they include both lignin and resistant starch. The difference are relatively small for many foods. Exceptions such as cornflakes are often cited, but these are the rare

Total dietary fibre (gravimetric)	Non-starch polysaccharides (NSP)	Non-cellulosic polysaccharides (NCP)	Other polysaccharides	Soluble fibre	Other sugar residues	Plant cell wall
					Uronic acids	
					Rhamnose	
			Pectin	– – – Arabinose		
				Xylose	
			Hemicellulose	– – –	Mannose	
				Insoluble fibre	Galactose	
		Cellulose	Cellulose		Glucose	
	Lignin	Lignin	Lignin		Lignin	
	Enzymically resistant starch					
	– –					
	Starch					

Figure 2.4
Diagram showing relationships between different ways of classifying and measuring the polysaccharides in foods. Broken lines indicate boundaries that are not absolute. (Modified from Asp and Johansson [1984]).

exceptions. In many cases the levels of precision of both methods, as obtained under routine conditions, are not sufficient to state that the values are significantly different.

———2.5———
SOURCES OF DIETARY FIBRE IN THE DIET

All plant foods contribute some dietary fibre to the diet but their relative importance differs according to the concentrations in the foods and the amounts eaten. There are in fact relatively few studies of dietary fibre intake in different populations, partly because of the lack of comprehensive data on the composition of the foods eaten in many countries, and also because of the difficulties inherent in the measurement of food consumption, which is one of the most difficult of nutritional techniques. This section will use primarily data on UK foods, supplemented with some compositional data from Sweden.

In the UK approximately 47% of the total fibre intake is derived from cereal foods, with similar amounts coming from white bread (14%) and high-extraction breads (16%), and the remainder from high-extraction breakfast cereals. About 38% is provided by vegetables and of this potatoes provide about one-third. Fruits provide around 8%, with the remaining fibre coming from a range of different foods including the small amounts of cereals often used in meat products and other processed foods (*Gregory et al., 1990*). The relative importance of the major groups – cereal foods, vegetables and fruits and nuts – is probably typical of most developed countries.

2.5.1 Cereals as Sources of Dietary Fibre

In most wholegrain cereals the seed coats are the major source of cell wall material. In the wheat grain the bran-rich outer layers, making up about 14% of the grain, contain 75% of the dietary fibre, whereas the endosperm, which is about 83% of the grain weight, contains only 24% of the dietary fibre. The amount of fibre provided by cereal products therefore depends very greatly on the extraction rate of the product. In wheat the dietary fibre content rises sharply once the extraction value exceeds 80%, from a value of around 2.5 g/100 g in 75% extraction to the value in the whole grain of around 12 g/100 g. Most of this increase occurs in the insoluble fractions because the soluble components are derived mainly from the endosperm walls. The composition of the dietary fibre is slightly different in the low extraction flours which have more galactose and mannose and virtually no lignin or uronic acids. In rye and barley the increase with extraction rate is not so steep and starts at around extraction rates of 65% or so; this is because the bran layers in these grains are more tightly fused to the grain. In both these cereals the concentrations of the soluble fractions do not change with extraction rate. The dietary fibre in rice rises steeply with extraction rate over 63%. In sorghum there is a progressive increase with extractions above 62%. These three cereals also show little or no increase in the soluble components with extraction. Table 2.5 gives some of the compositional data for these cereals derived from the TDF and NSP methods. In general the major non-cellulosic polysaccharides in wheat, rye and maize are arabinoxylans; in barley and oats the beta-glucans are also important. In rice the whole grain contains xylans with a low proportion of arabinose. The arabinans extracted from cereals possess very high water-binding capacities and these pentosans have been used to improve the breadmaking qualities of flours. In wheat they are insoluble, but soluble components are present in rye and barley. The

Table 2.5 Dietary fibre values in some cereals

Cereal (% extraction)	(g/100 g dry weight)				
	TDF	NSP	Sol NSP	Insol NSP	Lignin
Wheat (66)	2.2	2.4	1.3	1.3	Neg
Wheat (100)	12.1	9.5	1.3	8.2	2.2
Wheat (100)	ND	9.8	2.3	7.5	ND
Rye (66)	7.5	6.8	3.8	3.0	0.3
Rye (100)	16.1	12.5	3.8	9.7	4.6
Rye (100)	ND	13.2	4.6	8.6	ND
Barley (66)	8.2	7.9	3.9	4.0	Neg
Barley (100)	18.8	15.9	3.9	12.0	3.5
Barley (whole)	ND	16.7	4.5	12.2	ND
Maize (fine)	3.9	4.1	>0.5	3.4	0.8
Maize (coarse)	9.3	8.0	>0.5	8.8	3.5
Maize (unspecified)	ND	5.6	0.9	4.7	ND
Rice (64)	0.7	1.1	0.5	0.6	Neg
Rice (100)	19.2	13.0	0.5	18.7	3.9
Rice (brown)	ND	2.2	Neg	2.2	ND

ND = not determined; Neg = unmeasurable levels
This table includes data obtained with an AOAC-type TDF method and the NSP method (where ND is shown under TDF). As one can see the results of the two methods are comparable. The NSP method gives higher proportions of soluble components due to the higher pH of extraction around 5.6.

beta-glucans of oats and barley form very viscous solutions and this property can be a disadvantage in animal feeding because it reduces food intake. In humans this viscous property may be a factor contributing to the mechanisms reducing serum cholesterol values in subjects with elevated values.

Most of the dietary fibre in cereals is insoluble and in the whole grain is associated with lignin. This lignification restricts the extent of fermentation in the large bowel so that the cereal fibres are more effective contributors to increasing faecal bulk (see Chapter 3).

2.5.2 Vegetables

Vegetables, as consumed, have relatively low concentrations of dietary fibre, primarily because of their high water content. Typical values for the total fibre content range between 2 and 3 g/100 g (Table 2.6). The concentrations are higher in the seed legumes and even higher in the mature dry seeds as purchased. In most vegetables the cell walls are relatively undifferentiated and so the walls are thin with lignin restricted to the low amounts of vascular tissues. The NCP are very soluble so that over half their content is extracted into hot water. These polysaccharides are rich in uronans and arabinogalactans. The uronans are usually low

Table 2.6 Dietary fibre values in some vegetables

Vegetable	Total NSP (dm)	Cell.	NCP	SNSP	INSP	Total NSP (fw)
Broccoli	28.8	10.0	18.8	14.4	14.4	3.0
Brussels sprouts	29.8	8.6	21.2	16.2	13.6	5.6
Cabbage, Savoy	27.9	8.8	19.1	14.9	13.0	3.7
Cauliflower	21.5	5.5	16.0	10.6	10.6	1.8
Potato, early	6.7	2.7	4.0	3.5	3.2	1.1
Potato, main	6.4	2.0	4.4	3.8	2.6	1.2
Carrots	19.5	6.4	13.1	11.4	8.1	2.4
Swede	35.8	14.5	21.3	16.5	19.3	3.4
Turnip	36.2	17.0	19.2	14.0	22.2	5.7
Beans, haricot	19.5	4.6	14.9	9.1	10.4	17.0
Beans, red kidney	18.2	4.4	13.8	8.0	10.2	15.2
Peas, fresh	20.9	12.1	8.2	5.9	15.0	2.9
Cucumber	15.6	6.9	8.7	6.0	9.6	0.5
Peppers	22.4	9.0	13.4	10.0	12.4	1.6
Tomato	18.8	7.5	11.3	7.4	11.4	1.1

NSP = non-starch polysaccharides; Cell. = cellulose; NCP = non-cellulosic polysaccharides; SNSP = soluble NSP; INSP = insoluble NSP; dm = dry matter basis; fw = fresh weight basis

methoxyl compounds and have low gelling capacity. Table 2.6 gives some values different types of vegetable.

2.5.3 Fruits

These are also relatively minor sources of dietary fibre, with the concentrations as consumed being even lower than those of vegetables because of the high water content of many fruits. The cell walls are thin and undifferentiated, with low amounts of lignified vascular tissues. The seeds within the fruits are often heavily lignified and therefore highly resistant to digestion. The NCP are mainly soluble and rich in uronans. In some species these are high-methoxy forms and have gel-forming properties, although it is doubtful whether this property is displayed in the intestinal contents. Table 2.7 gives some typical values for different fruits.

——2.6——
SUMMARY OF THE PROPERTIES OF DIETARY FIBRE

As will be evident from the above, it is difficult to generalize about the properties of dietary fibre. In fact it is very naive to make a statement of the kind 'dietary fibre has the following properties' without specifying the

Table 2.7 Dietary fibre values in some fruits

Fruit	Total NSP (dm)	Cell.	NCP	SNSP	INSP	Total NSP (fw)
Apples	12.5	5.2	7.3	5.4	7.1	1.7
Bananas	4.5	1.0	3.5	2.8	1.7	1.1
Blackcurrants	16.5	3.5	13.0	7.5	9.0	3.6
Cherries	6.4	1.2	5.2	3.9	2.5	1.2
Grapes	3.4	1.2	2.2	1.7	1.7	0.6
Melon, honeydew	6.8	3.3	3.5	2.7	4.1	0.3
Oranges	15.0	3.4	11.6	9.8	5.2	2.2
Peach	13.5	3.9	9.6	7.1	6.4	1.5
Pears	15.8	4.7	11.1	5.1	10.7	2.4
Pineapple	9.1	3.9	5.2	0.8	8.3	1.2
Plums	11.2	2.1	9.1	7.5	3.7	1.8
Raspberry	21.5	9.7	11.8	5.9	6.8	2.5
Strawberry	11.9	4.1	7.8	5.1	6.8	1.4

NSP = non-starch polysaccharides; Cell. = cellulose; NCP = non-cellulosic polysaccharides; SNSP = soluble NSP; INSP = insoluble NSP; dm = dry matter basis; fw = fresh weight basis

source of the dietary fibre in some detail. However, we can advance some general principles, as follows:

1. Dietary fibre is derived from the plant cell walls in foods, with, in developed countries, some minor contributions from isolated polysaccharide additives used in processed foods.

2. The major components of dietary fibre are non-alpha-linked glucans or NSP. These are not hydrolysed by the endogenous secretions of the mammalian digestive tract and are, by definition, indigestible in the small intestine These resistant polysaccharides pass into the large intestine substantially unaltered, but undergo fermentation to a varying extent.

3. Some of the components of dietary fibre are water-soluble under the conditions prevailing in the small intestine, and some of these soluble polysaccharides are capable of increasing the viscosity of the contents of the intestine.

4. The insoluble components are often associated with lignin and other polyphenolic components which make the tissues containing them hydrophobic and resistant to fermentation. The complex lipids cutin and suberin have similar effects.

5. The measurement of dietary fibre requires techniques that provide an index of the plant cell walls in foods. This can be achieved by measuring the NSP, preferably in combination with an independent measurement of lignin. Indirect estimates

can be obtained by measuring the indigestible residue in the foods since in most foods this approximates to the plant cell wall material.

FURTHER READING

Asp N-G, Schweizer TF, Southgate, DAT, Theander, O. Dietary fibre analysis. In: *Dietary Fibre: A Component of Food*. Schweizer TF, Edwards CA eds. 1992, London: Springer Verlag, pp 57–101.

Englyst HN, Bingham SA, Runswick SS, Collinson E, Cummings JH. Dietary fibre (non-starch polysaccharides) in fruit, vegetables and nuts. *J Hum Nutr Dietet* 1998; 1: 247–86.

Englyst HN, Bingham SA, Runswick SA, Collinson E, Cummings JH. Dietary fibre (non-starch polysaccharides) in cereal products. *J Hum Nutr Dietet* 1989; 2: 253–71.

Nyman M, Siljestrom M, Pedersen B, Bach Knudsen KE, Asp N-G, Johansson C-G, Eggum BO. Dietary fiber content and composition in six cereals at different extraction rates. *Cereal Chemistry* 1984; 61: 14–19.

Paul AA, Southgate, DAT. *McCance and Widdowson's The Composition of Foods*, 4th ed. London: HMSO

Prosky L, DeVries J. *Controlling Dietary Fiber in Food Products*. New York: Van Nostrand Reinhold, 1992.

Selvendran RR, O'Neill MA. Isolation and analysis of cell walls from plant material. *Methods of Biochemical Analysis*, vol 32. Glick D, ed. New York: John Wiley, 1987, pp 25–145.

Southgate DAT. *Determination of Food Carbohydrates*. 2nd ed. London: Elsevier Applied Science Publishers.

Effects of Fibre and Resistant Starch on Intestinal Motility and Function

The basic premise of the dietary fibre hypothesis is that the populations of industrialized Western countries suffer from a form of chronic malnutrition. Within a few years of its inception this rather surprising idea had captured the imagination of the general public, clinicians, research workers and, in the present context most importantly, biomedical research funding agencies on both sides of the Atlantic. Nevertheless it has been extremely difficult to test the dietary fibre hypothesis directly. Although recommended intakes for fibre are now routinely included in the dietary guidelines of all developed nations, it has not yet been possible to confirm a protective role for fibre consumption in the aetiology of any disease. This is partly because scientific theories, by their very nature, can be refuted but never finally proven, and partly because the development of non-infectious diseases such as cancer, heart disease and diabetes occurs over many years. A direct test of the dietary fibre hypothesis is greatly hampered by the impossibility of controlling, or even measuring with any accuracy, the dietary habits of large numbers of people over such lengthy periods of time.

In spite of these difficulties, a great deal of indirect evidence has been acquired. The hypothesis is based on a set of propositions concerning the behaviour and effects of cell wall polysaccharides in the small intestine during digestion, and in the large bowel during the formation and passage of faeces. The physiological effects of cell wall polysaccharides have now been extensively explored in both human beings and laboratory animals, and a great deal of new knowledge about the biology of the gut has been generated. It is now well established that cell wall polysaccharides and resistant starch can affect the functioning of the entire alimentary tract, and thereby modify many of the metabolic processes in which the intestinal organs play a central role. However, it has also become evident that these various polysaccharides differ greatly in their biological and physical properties. Many of the original generalizations about the benefits of dietary fibre for human health were based on inadequate analytical data and a poor understanding of cell wall chemistry. The dietary fibre hypothesis has therefore had to be extensively modified in the light of emerging knowledge.

In this chapter the physiological effects of dietary fibre will be reviewed. As we have seen, the common characteristic of the various substances that are classified as dietary fibre and resistant starch is their ability to resist hydrolysis by digestive enzymes. As digestion and absorption progress, the fats, proteins and digestible carbohydrates disappear from the digesta, leaving the resistant polysaccharides behind in the gut lumen. As a result, the physical properties of the residual gut contents tend to reflect those of the cell wall polysaccharides which they contain. Food residues move through the alimentary canal under the influence of precisely controlled muscular contractions. One important outcome of the dietary fibre hypothesis has been the new light thrown on gastrointestinal motility and its relationship to the physical properties of food materials. Most of the effects observed have been benign or neutral in relation to health but, as we will see, some adverse effects of fibre have been reported, including occasional complete obstruction of the various organs of the alimentary canal.

It should now be clear that cell wall polysaccharides are the structural elements of plant foods, and they confer upon them physical character-istics including texture and viscosity. From the outset, the founders of the dietary fibre hypothesis were concerned mainly with the distinctive prop-erties of the raw, 'whole', unrefined or only lightly processed foods eaten in non-industrialized agrarian societies such as Africa and parts of the Far East, in contrast to the often highly processed cereal foods that character-ize Western diets. Surgeon Captain Cleave regarded processed cereals as the underlying cause of the syndrome he called the 'saccharine disease'. As Kenneth Heaton (1990) has pointed out, Cleave's original ideal can be neatly summed up in his borrowing of the phrase 'what God has joined together let no man put asunder'. Reading Cleave's work today, one wonders how he might have regarded the advent of manufactured food products to which fibre supplements had been added during processing. The implications of these two quite different approaches to the concept of dietary fibre will emerge repeatedly in this and later chapters.

—3.1—
THE ALIMENTARY TRACT: TRANSIT, DIGESTION, ABSORPTION

The alimentary tract comprises a highly integrated system of hollow organs which are adapted for the ingestion, digestion and absorption of nutrients. The gross anatomy of the human alimentary canal is illustrated in Fig. 3.1. For digestion and absorption to be performed effectively, the ingested food must be propelled from one compartment of the gut to the next at a rate that ensures that each step in the assimilation of nutrients is completed in an orderly manner. This is accomplished by the special-ized motor activities of the intestinal musculature. The intestinal wall contains two main layers of smooth muscle, with their fibres running in circular and longitudinal directions respectively. A third, thinner layer of muscle fibres, the muscularis mucosae, lies within the mucosa beneath the villi, and still finer fibres extend from this layer toward the tip of each villus. Electrical activity propagates throughout the layers of smooth muscle in the form of both slow waves and spikes. Together, these signals trigger waves of rhythmic contraction. Peristalsis, as this spontaneous muscular activity is called, is an intrinsic function of the alimentary tract

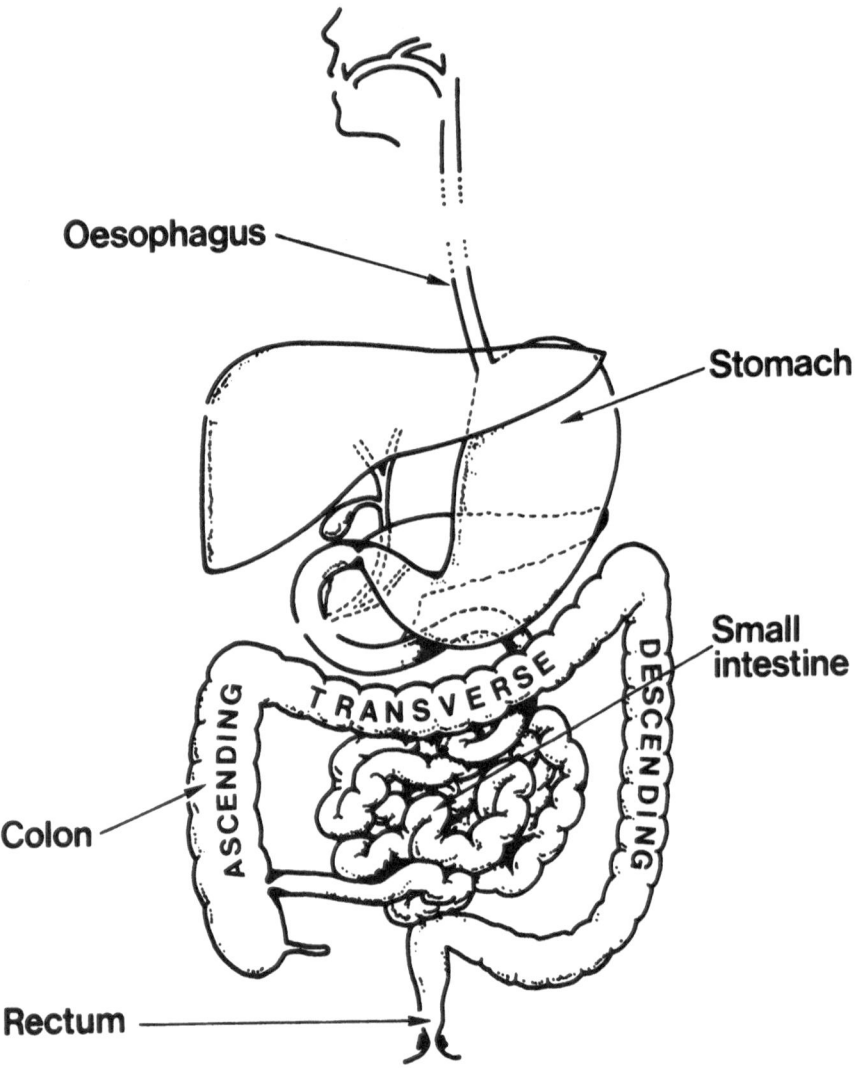

Figure 3.1
The general anatomy of the human alimentary tract.

which persists even in segments of intestine isolated *in vitro*. However, in the functioning gut, the intensity and frequency of peristalsis is regulated by the enteric nervous system, which is a neural network lying between the muscle layers, and by peptide hormones released by nutrients in the gut lumen.

Soon after it is eaten, food passes rapidly through the pharynx and oesophagus to the stomach, where it undergoes a prolonged process of disruption and stirring in the presence of hydrochloric acid and the gastric digestive enzymes. The semiliquid, partially digested food residue or chyme is ejected from the stomach at a controlled rate into the proximal part of the small intestine, where most nutrients are rapidly absorbed. Passage through the entire length of the small bowel to the colon takes a few hours but the period of retention in the large bowel is highly variable and under some degree of conscious control. The passage of digesta from one organ to another is regulated by the opening of muscular valves or sphincters at the gastric pylorus, the ileocaecal junction and the anus. The integration of all the various endocrine and neural signals from the olfactory organs, from the mucosal chemoreceptors, and from stretch-receptors in the muscle layer, ensures that peristalsis achieves an orderly combination of mixing and propulsive movements. Under normal circumstances we remain largely unaware of the activities of our own alimentary organs. The complex neuroendocrine system of the gut is largely independent of the central nervous system with which it shares many organizational characteristics, and it may be regarded almost as a 'brain' in its own right.

———3.2———
THE FIRST STAGES OF DIGESTION: PHARYNX AND OESOPHAGUS

The presence of NSP influences the physical properties of the gut contents at all levels in the alimentary tract, but the retention of an intact cellular structure in plant foods, and the textural characteristics that are associated with it, are most obviously experienced during mastication. Put at its simplest, hard foods have to be chewed more thoroughly before they can be swallowed. This alters the rate of food ingestion and, in all probability, increases the average size of the food particles passing through the oesophagus to the stomach. The most extreme example perhaps is the contrast between comminuted and whole raw fruit. Apples take longer to eat than juice takes to drink, and the eventual absorption of sugar into the bloodstream is much slower (*Haber et al., 1977*). This principle extends to other carbohydrate foods. It has been shown that, when healthy subjects are asked to swallow cubes of potato without chewing, the rate at which the starch is digested and absorbed is much slower than when they are allowed to chew *ad libitum* (*Read et al., 1986*). It is entirely probable that the available carbohydrates in hard and intractable plant foods are assimilated more slowly than their processed counterparts, simply because they are more difficult to eat quickly. However, this point has not been rigorously tested, and it is probably of little relevance to Western diets.

3.2.1 Oesophageal Obstruction

Under normal circumstances, food passes rapidly through the oesophagus, which has no digestive function. An obstruction of the oesophagus can occur during the ingestion of any type of food in patients with an *oesophageal stricture*, which is an acquired narrowing of the lumen usually located near the junction with the stomach. A blockage here, or at a higher level, may also be the first sign of the presence of an oesophageal tumour. As we shall later see, clinical interest in the use of soluble NSP for the control of metabolic diseases has led to the development of a variety of pharmaceutical products based upon very viscous NSP. One of the most common constituents is guar gum in the form of dry powder or granules, and often this is also the main constituent of patent 'medicines', pills and other preparations marketed as so-called slimming aids. In the early 1980s, isolated reports began to appear in the medical literature describing obstruction, and even rupture, of the oesophagus after ingestion of products containing guar gum.

It would appear that in most of the early cases of obstruction the material had usually been misused to the extent that it was ingested in a dry state. Powdered or granulated guar gum tends to become sticky when moistened so that on contact with saliva it may easily become lodged in the oesophagus, and then expand during hydration (*Ahlman, 1982; Edstrom & Petterson, 1982*). Pharmaceutical preparations containing guar granules are now marketed with clear instructions that the material should be hydrated before consumption, or sprinkled onto a substantial quantity of food. However, isolated cases of oesophageal obstruction due to guar gum have continued to appear in the literature. In recent cases the cause appears most frequently to have been products designed to assist in weight reduction, and the patients have usually had a history of oesophageal abnormalities (*Henry et al., 1986; Morse & Malloy, 1990;*

Opper et al., 1990; Seidner et al., 1990; Halama & Mauldin, 1992). So-called 'diet pills' containing cellulose have also been reported as a cause of total obstruction of the distal oesophagus in patients with previously undiagnosed oesophageal stricture *(Jones & Pillsbury, 1990).*

Although conventional foods with a high fibre content seem no more likely than any other kind of food to cause acute obstruction of the healthy oesophagus, pharmaceutical products and patent medicines or 'health foods' containing high levels of isolated NSP evidently carry some risks, albeit mainly to subjects with underlying oesophageal disease. Symptomless oesophageal stricture is relatively common, particularly in the elderly, and this problem must be taken into account by those developing high-fibre products. In the USA the Food and Drug Administration (FDA) has expressed concern that products containing guar gum may cause choking, and in 1990 it recommended a ban on diet products based on guar. Under a voluntary agreement proposed at the time of writing in 1993, two American health food manufacturers agreed to 'resolve the concerns' of 11 of the states, and to recall and destroy all diet products containing more than 0.5% guar gum. Under the proposals, higher levels of guar gum would be permitted in bulk laxatives, but only if labelled in accordance with FDA regulations.

——3.3——
THE GASTRIC PHASE

Although the human stomach is essentially a muscular sac with few obvious internal structures, it does contain functionally specialized compartments. During ingestion of a meal, food accumulates in the gastric fundus and body. At this stage, muscular activity is relatively quiescent, and the walls of the stomach stretch to accommodate the increased volume. When the stomach is full, more pronounced mechanical activity begins. Waves of tonic contraction begin to flow from the body toward the antrum. These relatively weak 'mixer waves' stir the masticated food with the acidic gastric juice, causing further reduction of particle size and assisting the initial hydrolysis of polymeric food constituents. In the antrum the muscular waves are stronger, and develop into contractile rings which force the antral contents toward the pylorus. The pyloric sphincter opens sufficiently to allow a relatively small quantity of material to pass into the duodenum, but the major fraction undergoes retrograde flow, backwards through the contractile ring, toward the gastric body. This vigorous movement assists in the further mechanical degradation of food particles. The rate of gastric emptying depends upon a balance between the resistance of the pyloric sphincter and the intensity of antral muscular activity. The functional compartmentation of the stomach leads to some segregation of partially digested food. During the course of a meal, solid particles are retained in the fundus, while liquids and finely suspended solids are preferentially emptied into the duodenum. The restrictive effect of the pyloric sphincter ensures that particles are retained in the stomach until the grinding effect of the antrum has reduced them to about 1–2 mm in size. This ensures that the duodenal contents have a texture which is optimal for digestion.

Perhaps the main reason for the striking effect of chewing on the digestibility of starchy foods is the role played by particle size in the control of gastric emptying. However, as we have seen, not all non-digestible polysaccharides are hard and fibrous. Pectins, beta-glucans, mucilages, exudate gums and chemically modified cellulose gums are all soluble in aqueous media under physiological conditions, and many become viscous as they are dispersed in the gastric lumen. Viscosity also appears to retard gastric emptying to some extent, and this factor plays some role as a determinant of the metabolic response to meals. Guar gum and isolated pectin both reduce the rate of gastric emptying, and increase the hydrostatic pressure within the antrum, probably by increasing the viscosity of the antral contents to an extent that slows the rate at which liquids can be expelled through the pylorus (*Meyer et al., 1986*). The result is a delay in the rate at which liquids enter the duodenum. At an early stage in the study of soluble dietary fibre and its effect on carbohydrate metabolism it was proposed that delayed gastric emptying was the principal physiological effect of guar gum (*Holt et al., 1979*) but, as we shall see, effects on small intestinal absorption have subsequently been shown to be more important.

3.3.1 Gastric Obstruction

Unlike the oesophagus, which has a small volume and plays no role in digestion, the stomach is specialized for temporary storage of food. It also produces copious secretions which can hydrate and liquify its contents. Acute obstruction of the stomach by poorly hydrated but soluble components of dietary fibre, such as guar gum, is therefore virtually impossible. However insoluble plant cell wall materials have been implicated in the formation of gastric phytobezoars. These structures are solid masses or concretions which form slowly and persist in the stomach indefinitely. Typically they are composed of undigested plant material, including whole seeds. Formation of a bezoar, with or without symptoms, is often a complication of partial gastrectomy or surgical destruction of the vagus nerve. If removal of the bezoar becomes necessary, surgery is usual, although the use of cellulase to degrade them without surgery has been described (*Stanten & Peters, 1975*). Again, it seems unlikely that the formation of gastric bezoars is a hazard for healthy individuals consuming conventional high-fibre foods but the use of specialized high-fibre products by patients with clinical abnormalities of the stomach may be unwise. In recent years NSP supplements have been added to liquid formula diets in order to maintain the morphology and function of the distal gut (*Scheppach et al., 1990*) but there have been reports which suggest that this may entail a risk of gastric bezoar formation in tube-fed patients (*McIvor et al., 1990*).

———3.4———
THE SMALL INTESTINE

The small intestine is the longest of the digestive organs and, as befits the principal site of nutrient absorption, it has the greatest surface area. Digestive enzymes, bile acids and water enter the lumen in the upper duodenum. Hydrolysis of the large digestible polymers in food – proteins, triglycerides and most of the starch – occurs rapidly within the first 2 m or so of duodenum and jejunum. The final hydrolysis of oligosaccharides and peptides occurs at the mucosal surface and the products are absorbed into the circulation via the specialized epithelial cells that line the intestinal mucosa. Much of the water and electrolytes secreted into the gut during digestion are also reabsorbed with the nutrients as the food residues progress along the small bowel.

As in the other organs of the alimentary tract, peristaltic activity in the small intestine has dual mixing and propulsive functions. During fasting and sleep, a cyclical pattern of muscular activity, the migrating myoelectric complex, moves through the small intestine toward the colon at more or less regular intervals. Distension of the intestinal wall by food interrupts this pattern and triggers concentric 'segmentation contractions' which lead to the formation of stationary contractile rings. These form and relax spontaneously several times per minute, mixing the intestinal contents as they do so. Peristaltic waves also occur, moving in a distal direction at around 1 cm per second, and rhythmic low-amplitude contractions of the villi have been observed in response to the presence of food or other chemical stimuli in the lumen. These various types of muscular activity ensure that the partially digested gut contents, or chyme, is well stirred, and conveyed along the intestine at about 1 cm per minute. Muscular activity is generally less well defined and less intense in the distal half of the small bowel, so that movement is slower and food residues tend to accumulate in the distal ileum before passage into the large bowel. In adult humans the first fermentable residues from a meal enter the colon approximately four and a half hours after ingestion.

3.4.1 Cell Wall Polysaccharides in the Small Intestine

Although the diverse group of polysaccharides which comprise dietary fibre are all resistant to hydrolysis by mammalian pancreatic enzymes, the complex, three-dimensional architecture of plant cell walls tends to be disrupted physically during mastication and the initial stages of digestion in the stomach. The insoluble components of cell walls will be degraded to fine particles, and the soluble polysaccharides will become dispersed in the aqueous phase of the gut contents. The susceptibility of cell walls to physical disruption during their passage through the alimentary tract varies considerably from one type of food to another. Any intact cell walls that survive the early stages of digestion will form a barrier separating digestive enzymes from their substrates. Even when enzymes and their substrates come into contact and hydrolysis is in progress, the presence of cell wall polysaccharides may slow the diffusion of hydrolytic products through the partially digested matrix in the gut lumen.

When an indigestible but rapidly fermented disaccharide sugar such as lactulose is taken by mouth, transit to the colon occurs about one and a half hours earlier than it does if the same dose of lactulose is added to a starchy meal. The presence of solid food residues evidently slows transit, probably by delaying gastric emptying and perhaps also by increasing the viscosity of the chyme so that it tends to resist the peristaltic flow. Moderate quantities of insoluble dietary fibre do not seem to delay transit any further, but supplements of highly viscous NSP such as guar gum and pectin have been shown to modify small intestinal motility and increase mouth to caecum transit time (*Bueno et al., 1981*). In the rat, most of this delay occurs in the stomach and in the terminal ileum (*Brown et al., 1988*).

3.4.2 Metabolic Effects of Dietary Fibre

Interest in the ability of plant cell walls and isolated components of dietary fibre to modify the motility and digestive functions of the small intestine stems largely from the proposed role of dietary fibre as a protective factor against metabolic diseases, and especially diabetes mellitus. Cleave's early premise that diabetes was but one aspect of a complex syndrome he termed the 'saccharine disease' was enthusiastically taken up and developed by Trowell, who surmised that insulin-independent diabetes was rare, if not non-existent, before the introduction of mechanized flour milling. The mechanism proposed to account for the protective effects of unrefined carbohydrate foods was that a diet in which they were predominant would favour the slow absorption and assimilation of glucose. This hypothesis has encouraged experimenters to measure the effects of cell wall polysaccharides on the absorption of carbohydrates from the small intestine, and to search for 'slow-release' or 'lente carbohydrate' foods, characterized by a low 'glycaemic index'.

3.4.3 The Glycaemic Index

The concept of the glycaemic index has developed from the glucose tolerance test, which is a clinical technique for evaluating glucose metabolism in humans. In healthy subjects the concentration of glucose in the blood is maintained within a normal range by the opposing actions of the pancreatic hormones insulin and glucagon. After a meal containing carbohydrates, glucose enters the circulation via the veins draining the intestinal mucosa. The rise in glucose concentration stimulates the production of gastrointestinal peptides, including insulin, which, among other effects, stimulates the uptake and utilization of glucose by the liver and peripheral tissues. The concentration of glucose in the blood then rapidly falls toward the normal fasting level of about 5 mmol/l. Any tendency to fall below this value is counteracted by the production of glucagon, which stimulates the release of glucose from endogenous sources. In diabetes mellitus the homeostatic control of glucose metabolism fails to function properly and the blood glucose concentration is abnormally high, either because insulin is not produced (insulin-dependent diabetes, IDDM) or because the tissues become resistant to its effects (non-insulin-dependent diabetes, NIDDM).

The glucose tolerance test is a procedure in which the changing concentration of glucose in the blood of an individual patient is measured following the consumption of a standard carbohydrate test meal (50 g of glucose in water). In a glycaemic index test, a group of healthy volunteers are fasted overnight and then each is given a test meal of the experimental food containing a standardized quantity of total carbohydrate. The concentration of glucose in the blood is then measured over a period of about 3 hours. The glycaemic index of each test food is the ratio calculated by dividing the area under the blood glucose curve following the test meal by that produced by an equal quantity of some reference food such as glucose or white bread. The final value is an average calculated for the group of subjects in order to allow for variation between individuals. This is a simple but effective experimental tool which has enabled the rate of glucose assimilation for different foods to be quantified and compared.

A list of glycaemic index values for some common foods, standardized against a 50 g dose of glucose, is given in Table 3.1. It is obvious that many of the foods with a low glycaemic index are pulses. This is probably because legume seeds have relatively thick cell walls which resist destruction during processing and cooking, and serve as a barrier which protects their starch content from hydrolysis during digestion. This type of effect of dietary fibre is very difficult to predict from analytical values of fibre alone because it is a function of the structural disposition of plant cell walls, rather than the absolute quantity of polysaccharides within the food. It should be noted that, although the glycaemic index has been advocated as a means to calculate the metabolic effects of complex diets for diabetics, its use for this purpose remains controversial.

Diets containing very high levels of dietary fibre derived primarily from legumes have been used in experimental studies with beneficial results (*Simpson et al., 1981*). However, the improvement in metabolic parameters has usually been accompanied by weight loss, which is also known to be a key factor in the management of diabetes. It is often difficult to identify a specific metabolic effect of dietary fibre, as distinct from the effects of reduced fat and energy consumption that accompany any major increase in fibre intake. It has been forcefully argued that the role of cell wall polysaccharides in the aetiology and management of

Table 3.1 Glycaemic Index Values For A Range of Foods[a]

Food	Glycaemic Index[b]
Cereal products	
Bread (white)	69 +/- 5
Bread (wholemeal)	72 +/- 6
Rice (white)	72 +/- 9
Rice (brown)	66 +/- 5
Spaghetti (white)	50 +/- 8
Spaghetti (wholemeal)	42 +/- 4
Cornflakes	80 +/- 6
Porridge oats	49 +/- 8
Vegetables	
Potato (new)	70 +/- 8
Potato (instant)	80 +/- 13
Beans (tinned baked)	40 +/- 3
Beans (butter)	36 +/- 4
Beans (haricot)	31 +/- 6
Beans (kidney)	29 +/- 8
Beans (soya)	15 +/- 5
Fruit	
Apples	39 +/- 3
Oranges	40 +/- 3
Banana	62 +/- 9
Sugars	
Glucose[c]	100
Fructose	20 +/- 5
Sucrose	59 +/- 10
Honey	87 +/- 8

a Data taken from Jenkins et al. (1981)
b Values are means and standard errors obtained from experiments with 5–10 subjects.
c Data was calculated from the area under the glucose response curve after eating a portion of food equivalent to 50 g of glucose, divided by the response to a 50 g dose of glucose.

diabetes has not been properly established, and that over-zealous use of high-fibre foods in the diabetic diet may not be justifiable (*Berger & Venhaus, 1992*).

Clearly, if a substantial proportion of the starch content of a food is chemically resistant to pancreatic amylase, its constituent glucose molecules will not be absorbed and can make no contribution to the glycaemic response. Retrograded amylose is extremely resistant to digestion *in vitro* (Fig 1.3) and this material passes through the small intestine to the colon. Relatively small amounts of retrograded amylose are found in conventional foods, although particular foods such as cooked peas which have been cooled and stored may contain appreciable quantities. Unripe bananas also contain chemically resistant starch as a natural constituent, and have an abnormally low glycaemic index as a result. Englyst and Cummings (*1988*) have proposed that dietary starches should be classified as 'rapidly digestible' (RDS) 'slowly digestible' (SDS) and 'resistant' (RS). The resistant starch fraction can be subdivided further into 'physically inaccessible starch' (RS1), 'resistant starch granules' such as those found in unripe bananas or raw potato (RS2) and 'retrograded starch' (RS3). The full nutritional implications of resistant starch are still under investigation by several research groups.

3.4.4 Isolated Polysaccharide Gums

In parallel with studies on the glycaemic effects of intact foods, a great deal of experimental work has also been carried out on isolated components of dietary fibre that could be used as dietary supplements or pharmaceutical preparations for the management of diabetes. David Jenkins and his colleagues, working at Oxford in the early 1970s, conducted much of the early work on the physiological effects of dietary fibre in the small bowel. They were able to demonstrate important effects of dietary fibre, although the use of glucose tolerance studies with human subjects made it difficult to be sure of the mechanisms underlying the observed effects. Many experiments were carried out using isolated components of fibre administered in combination with a liquid test meal containing glucose. It soon emerged that under these conditions only soluble polysaccharides with a high viscosity led to a significant reduction in postprandial glycaemia. Wheat bran, which is the major source of dietary fibre in wholemeal wheat products, was ineffective (*Jenkins et al., 1978*). This was a very important finding because it showed that one of the most readily available sources of fibre in Western diets was of little significance in the management of diabetes. Moreover, it did not lend any support to Trowell's contention that diabetes mellitus only appeared in the West with the introduction of modern cereal processing technology. Nevertheless the findings provoked considerable interest in what soon came to be called 'soluble dietary fibre', and in one polysaccharide, guar gum, in particular.

Guar gum is derived from the cluster bean (*Cyamopsis tetragonoloba*), a legume that is native to eastern Asia. Unlike most components of dietary fibre, guar gum is a storage polysaccharide rather than a component of the cell wall. It has a high viscosity in water and is widely used as a food additive for controlling texture and emulsion stability in products such as soups and ice cream. However, dietary intakes from these sources are relatively trivial. The quantities that proved to be effective when incorporated into experimental meals ranged from about 3 to 20 g. At these levels the test meals became extremely viscous, and some workers argued that the main physiological effect of guar gum, and other viscous polysaccharides such as pectin, was to slow gastric emptying, thus reducing the rate at which glucose entered the small bowel (*Holt et al., 1979*). The alternative proposal was that guar acted primarily in the small bowel itself. This issue has remained a matter of some controversy, and it is of practical importance because of the implications for the design of products containing guar gum. For example, if the mechanism of action depends upon a high viscosity in the stomach, then any product intended to be added to food must be made to undergo hydration before, or very soon after, ingestion. The weight of evidence now suggests that the proximal small intestine is the major site at which viscous polysaccharides such as guar gum, beta-glucan and some viscous forms of pectin, influence the rate of nutrient digestion and absorption (*Blackburn et al., 1984*).

Under normal conditions, glucose, amino acids and peptides, and fatty acids are all absorbed rapidly by the mucosal cells that line the surfaces of the proximal small bowel. This high rate of absorption tends to dissipate the concentration of nutrients in the fluid environment immediately adjacent to the villi, and unless this substrate is replaced by movement from the bulk phase, the total flux of nutrients tends to decline. The intestinal lumen is normally well stirred by the peristaltic movements of the muscular gut wall and so mixing of the fluid layers serves to replace the absorbed material. However, this process becomes much less efficient when the viscosity of the luminal contents is high. Both propulsive movements and stirring are reduced and under these circumstances mixing becomes less efficient, and diffusion becomes the predominant mechanism conveying nutrients through the boundary fluid layers to the mucosal surface. However, diffusion is a relatively slow process, and intraluminal transport becomes an increasingly important rate-limiting step in nutrient absorption and assimilation.

The high viscosity of water-soluble polysaccharides is caused by weak interactions within the dispersed network of carbohydrate polymers. In theory the presence of these polymers in the fluid environment of the gut lumen could restrict the diffusion of nutrient molecules. In practice, however, at low polymer concentrations, they seem to impose relatively little restriction on the diffusion of low molecular weight solutes. This is probably not true, though, in the case of lipid micelles derived from digestion of dietary fats. These very large molecular aggregates containing fatty acids, bile salts and cholesterol diffuse from the site of fat hydrolysis in the gut lumen to the mucosal surface. Diffusion of micelles is slowed by polysaccharide gums independently of any effect of viscosity on stirring, and this effect contributes to the delayed absorption of fat and cholesterol. The ability of guar gum to slow the intestinal absorption of cholesterol from mixed micelles is illustrated in Fig. 3.2.

As nutrient absorption is slowed, so the process is extended in time, and displaced physically along the length of the small bowel. This reduces the rate at which nutrients appear in the circulation, and increases the exposure of the gut surface to nutrients. In experimental animals these effects may trigger the release of regulatory hormones, and stimulate the growth of mucosal cells.

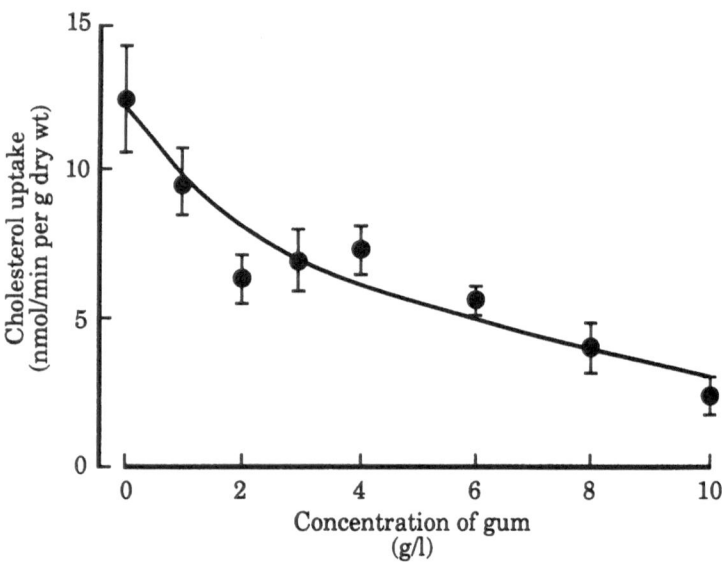

Figure 3.2
Cholesterol absorption from a mixed micellar suspension, by isolated everted sacs of rat intestine exposed to increasing concentrations of oat gum in the bathing medium. (Reproduced from Lund et al. [1989] with the permission of the British Journal of Nutrition.*)*

The discovery that viscous polysaccharides can improve the postprandial glycaemic response in diabetics has led to the development of various pharmaceutical products containing guar gum. As was mentioned earlier, these products can be added to food or taken with meals in the form of a drink, and they can assist in the management of those diabetic patients who find them palatable and acceptable for prolonged use. Guar has also been added successfully to bread in large enough quantities to ensure that an ingested bolus becomes very viscous in the stomach and small intestine, and the digestion and absorption of starch from such products is markedly slower than from conventional bread. However the product is expensive to produce and does not appear to be widely used at the time of writing. Few Western foods contain viscous polysaccharides at high enough levels to make much difference to intraluminal viscosity, but oats, which are rich in beta-glucan gum, are one important exception. Other foods, including legumes such as beans and lentils, also have a relatively low 'glycaemic index' but, although this has often been assumed to be due to the presence of viscous or so-called 'gel-forming' polysaccharides, the varieties of legumes common in Western diets are not rich in such substances. The slow digestion of legume starch appears to be due primarily to the survival of cell walls after cooking.

3.4.5 Binding Effects in the Small Intestine

Many cell wall polysaccharides, and associated lignin polymers, have charged groups that can interact with ionized species in the aqueous phase of the gut contents. Such interactions can, at least in theory, restrict the bioavailability of nutrients for transport by the cells of the intestinal mucosa. Iron, zinc and calcium are relatively poorly absorbed from the human diet. The limiting factor is usually the formation of insoluble precipitates or non-absorbable complexes in the intestinal lumen. Various forms of dietary fibre have been observed to bind metal ions *in vitro*, and it has often been stated that the consumption of diets rich in unrefined cereals might lead to a general reduction in the bioavailability of mineral nutrients. This concern is probably the most commonly proposed adverse effect of dietary fibre, both in the scientific and the popular literature, and because of this the topic will be dealt with in some detail in the next chapter.

Intraluminal binding of organic nutrients and bile acids has also been received a great deal of attention from researchers. The main reason for this is that it has seemed to provide a mechanism to explain yet another aspect of the dietary fibre hypothesis, the proposed protective effect of dietary fibre against heart disease. Some NSP have been shown substantially to reduce plasma cholesterol levels in man, at least under experimental conditions. The most effective material appears to be pectin, but other sources of fibre such as oat beta-glucan, ispaghula husk and even modified cellulose gums have been identified as potentially hypocholesterolaemic. In a recent (*1992*) review, Truswell and Beynen have estimated that about 10 g of pectin must be consumed each day to lower the plasma total cholesterol by 5–10%. It would necessitate the consumption of about 1 kg of fruit and vegetables if this level of pectin were to be derived from natural sources alone.

The mechanism underlying the effect of dietary fibre on plasma cholesterol is still unclear, and the problem has prompted many studies on the effects of fibre on bile acid absorption. Bile acids are natural surfactants that are synthesized from cholesterol in the liver, and released from the gall bladder into the small intestinal lumen. Although bile salts participate in the emulsification of fat and the formation of micelles, they are not absorbed in the proximal small intestine, but instead they are taken up by an efficient active transport system in the distal ileum, near the junction with the colon. From here they are returned to the liver via the portal bloodstream and resecreted into the proximal small intestine, typically within the duration of a single meal. The enterohepatic circulation of bile salts can be interrupted by the consumption of artificial sequestrants such as ion-exchange resins, which prevent reabsorption and lead to increased faecal excretion. This leads to a drain on the body's cholesterol resources, a shift in hepatic cholesterol metabolism towards bile salt synthesis and eventually to a reduction in serum cholesterol. This principle is used clinically to treat some forms of hypercholesterolaemia.

Some sources of dietary fibre have been shown to bind bile acids *in vitro*. The pioneering work on this topic by Eastwood and his colleagues led to the proposal that dietary fibre may act as a natural bile acid sequestrant (*Eastwood, 1969*) but, although this hypothesis is well established in the literature, it has never been proven conclusively. Indeed, the balance of evidence suggests that it is not an important mechanism influencing human cholesterol metabolism. This conclusion is based partly on the fact that the most effective hypocholesterolaemic polysaccharides are pectin, guar gum and oat beta-glucan, which are relatively poor bile acid sequestrants. On the other hand, highly lignified, largely insoluble tissues, such as wheat bran, are effective bile acid sequestrants *in vitro*, but they have been shown conclusively not to reduce plasma cholesterol in humans. Moreover, the maximum binding of bile acids occurs at acid pH, whereas the contents of the distal ileum where bile salts are actively absorbed are usually at near-neutral pH. Viscous polysaccharides probably modify cholesterol metabolism by reducing cholesterol absorption in the proximal small intestine, and perhaps by inhibiting bile salt uptake in the distal ileum by the mechanisms discussed earlier in this chapter (*Lund et al., 1989*).

Aside from cholesterol metabolism, the intraluminal binding of bile salts and other organic molecules may have important physiological effects. Bile salts have been shown to stimulate colonic contractions and fluid secretion, so one possibility is that they are released into the large bowel and act as a kind of natural laxative. Other, possibly adverse effects of bile salts in the colon will be considered in Chapter 5.

In healthy human subjects, the consumption of diets rich in dietary fibre has been shown to cause an increase in the faecal excretion of lipids and protein. A substantial proportion of this material appears to be derived from dietary fat and proteins that have escaped digestion, perhaps as a result of sequestration by cell wall polysaccharides, but a large fraction is of endogenous origin. There is little evidence that these minor faecal nutrient losses are of much nutritional significance in prosperous societies, but they probably reflect changes in intestinal growth and function which may have consequences for health (see Chapter 4).

3.4.6 Obstruction in the Small Intestine

Under normal circumstances viscous non-starch polysaccharide gums will be well hydrated by the time they enter the duodenum. Mastication and gastric motility reduce even coarse food to fine particles, and the highly efficient peristaltic activity of the small intestine is well adapted to overcome resistance to propulsion. We might therefore expect blockage of the small bowel by foods rich in dietary fibre to be a rare event. This seems generally to be true, but isolated incidents involving obstruction have been reported in the clinical literature. In most cases the immediate cause seems to have been wheat or oat bran cereals consumed at levels very significantly above the normal range. The patients have usually been rather elderly, with a history of abdominal surgery (*Cooper & Tracey, 1989; Rosario et al., 1990*). However, Allen-Mersh and De Jode (*1982*) described an elderly man with no surgical history who ate two helpings of a bran cereal at breakfast time and developed intestinal obstruction by evening. The obstruction occurred in the distal ileum and had to be removed by direct surgical access to the small bowel lumen. McClurken and Carp (1988) described a similar case involving a middle-aged man, again with no previous abdominal surgery, who also developed complete small intestinal obstruction after eating two bowls of bran cereal. Again, the obstruction, which was vividly described by the authors as an 'inspissated toothpaste-like plug', had to be removed surgically.

In general, although dietary fibre eaten as a component of ordinary unprocessed foods does modify small intestinal motility to some extent, the effects are probably beneficial. However, attempts to exploit the beneficial effects of fibre, either by the fabrication of very enriched foods or the use of pharmaceutical supplements, can lead to a risk of obstruction in susceptible individuals, particularly where they consume unusually large quantities. Meiser et al. (1990) have recently described a series of 73 patients with intermittent incomplete intestinal obstruction, 52 of whom had a history of previous abdominal surgery. There was no particular investigation of the role of dietary fibre in this study, but intake of 'bulky food' during the previous 12–48 hours was judged to be a precipitating factor in 47 of the patients. It would seem then that for a few patients, most of whom are probably identifiable from their medical history, intake of dietary fibre should be restricted, to the extent that only a modest fraction of the daily allowance is obtained from any one meal or food source.

------3.5------
EFFECTS ON THE FUNCTION OF THE LARGE BOWEL

The functions of the colon are to salvage endogenous materials shed into the gut lumen, to recover food residues that have escaped digestion and absorption in the small bowel, and to form and store faeces. The motility of the large intestine, though similar in principle to that of the rest of the alimentary tract, has its own specialized characteristics. In general, propulsion is slower, but mixing is very thorough. The longitudinal muscle fibres of the colon are localized into three distinct bands, the tineae coli. Contraction of the circular fibres occurs in localized rings. The combined contractile activity of these muscle layers causes the intermediate segments of colonic wall to stretch and bulge outward to form bag-like haustrations between the rings. These localized, stationary or slowly migrating contractions are similar to the segmentation contractions of the small bowel. The contractile rings intrude deeply into the colonic lumen, stirring the faecal contents and exposing it thoroughly to the mucosal surface, which is specialized for water absorption. The high viscosity of the faecal material necessitates particularly powerful musculature to achieve this, and leads to relatively high pressures within the colonic lumen.

The importance of cell wall polysaccharides as the natural means of increasing faecal bulk and stool frequency was one of the original tenets of the dietary fibre hypothesis as formulated by Burkitt and others, and this is still perhaps the most widely recognized physiological property of dietary fibre. As we have seen earlier, the benefits of 'roughage' were widely recognized before the twentieth century, but the originality of the fibre hypothesis lay in the concept of chronic constipation as a virtually universal condition in industrialized societies, and in the great variety of diseases which were thought to stem from this condition. Burkitt and others proposed a series of hypothetical mechanisms to explain the aetiology of many diseases of the large bowel, and some conditions that are perhaps less obviously associated with the gastrointestinal tract. Central to the hypothesis was the idea that constipation leads to both an undesirably high intracolonic pressure and prolonged straining at stool. It was proposed that the chronic physical stresses associated with these high pressures caused degenerative changes in the colorectal wall and also in the large veins of the lower abdomen and legs, eventually giving rise to diseases such as haemorrhoids, colonic diverticulae and varicose veins. Furthermore, it was suggested that slow transit of faecal material through the colon and rectum created conditions favouring the development of cancer.

3.5.1 Colonic Microflora

The formation of faeces and the control of defecation are functions associated with the left or descending colon. The caecum and the right colon harbour a rich microbial flora commonly containing over 500 bacterial species. The colonic environment is poorly supplied with nutrients, and unabsorbed dietary carbohydrates provide most of the substrates for growth and metabolism of the intracolonic flora. This substantial bacterial mass undoubtedly makes an important contribution to human physiology. It is known that the colonic microflora helps to salvage unabsorbed organic materials, and makes their energy content at least partly available to the host (*Livesey, 1992*); it contributes to the factors controlling the renewal of the epithelial cells lining the alimentary tract; and it modulates the immune system in subtle ways. Nevertheless the details of these functions are imperfectly understood at present. It has been suggested that the colonic bacterial mass should be looked upon as a single metabolic entity, or even as an organ in its own right. One important side-effect of the dietary fibre hypothesis has been to stimulate interest in this problem and increase our knowledge of human colonic microbiology.

The faecal microorganisms degrade many components of dietary fibre, as well as undigested starch, to yield the volatile fatty acids butyrate, propionate and acetate which are transported into and across the colonic mucosa. Butyrate functions as a substrate for the growth and metabolism of the colonic mucosal cells. Propionate and acetate are absorbed and metabolized by the liver, and up to three-quarters of the caloric value of the NSP becomes available to the body by these routes. The other major breakdown products of carbohydrate fermentation are hydrogen, methane and carbon dioxide, which together comprise flatus gas. The total volume of flatus produced by individuals varies considerably, as does its tendency to cause unpleasant symptoms of distension and abdominal pain. Some subjects report discomfort and flatulence when consuming high-fibre diets, but much of this may be caused by fermentation of low molecular weight carbohydrates, and particularly the poorly digestible oligosaccharides such as stachyose and verbascose that are often present in high concentrations in fibre-rich foods such as legume seeds.

Starch that escapes hydrolysis in the small intestine will also be available for fermentation in the colon, but not all of the starch fractions mentioned earlier are equally susceptible. This issue is still under investigation but it appears that, while RS1 and RS2 are rapidly and completely fermented by the colonic microflora, some forms of RS3 (retrograded amylose) are fermented much more slowly. Indeed, a small fraction of retrograded amylose prepared from maize starch is recoverable in the faeces of rats. The physiological consequences of such differences in starch metabolism remain an important issue for further research.

3.5.2 Faecal Output

The mildly laxative properties of wheat bran have been recognized since the time of Hippocrates (*c.* 460–377 BC), whose writings suggest that he was aware of its usefulness in the treatment of constipation. During the nineteenth and early twentieth centuries a number of medical authorities advocated the consumption of wholemeal cereals. Cereal products were particularly popular in the USA, where JH Kellogg prescribed wholegrain diets for his patients at the Battle Creek Sanatorium, and Sylvester Graham developed 'Graham crackers'. The emergence of the dietary fibre hypothesis in the latter years of this century had been preceded in the thirties by experimental studies with human subjects undertaken to quantify the effects of wheat bran on faecal output.

The composition of faeces is complex. In healthy individuals the water content is fairly constant at about 75%. Around one-third of the dry mass is composed of a mixture of viable microorganisms and bacterial cell debris. The organic constituents comprise cellulose and other polysaccharides, protein, about half of which is bacterial in origin, and fat. In healthy individuals less than 10 g of fat is excreted per day, but this quantity is increased if there is any deficiency in liver function. There are also a number of excreted organic compounds, which, although they account for only a small fraction of the faecal dry weight, do determine many of the properties of faeces. The characteristic colour is provided largely by modified bile pigments, the most important of which is stercobilin, a bacterial metabolite of bilirubin. The odour is due to indole, scatole, hydrogen sulphide and other bacterial metabolites. The remaining dry bulk is composed of undigested food residues, a component that can vary from almost zero to several tens of grams per day, depending upon the diet. Most of this material consists of NSP and, under certain circumstances, resistant starch.

Wheat bran is a largely insoluble, highly lignified plant tissue, which resists fermentation in the colon, and so increases faecal dry matter. Most importantly, however, it resists the re-absorption of faecal water during transit through the bowel, so that the moisture content of the faeces is also increased by its presence. The increment in stool mass caused by wheat bran depends to some extent on particle size, but in healthy Western populations it has been shown that, for every 1 g of wheat bran consumed per day, the output of stool is increased by between 3 and 5 g. Many other sources of dietary fibre also have this property of water retention. For example ispaghula, which is a mucilaginous material derived from Psyllium and containing a high proportion of non-fermentable polysaccharides, is used pharmaceutically as a bulk laxative. However, not all forms of dietary fibre contribute significantly to faecal bulk. Polysaccharides such as pectin, guar and oat beta-glucan are readily fermented by anaerobic bacteria, and are therefore decomposed during transit through the colon. The overall effect of such materials on faecal mass depends upon their contribution to bacterial growth.

Clearly the susceptibility of NSP to microbial fermentation somewhat complicates their effects on faecal bulk. As mentioned in the previous section, unfermented fibre contributes to both the dry weight and moist bulk of faeces. Fermentation of NSP will reduce its mass and modify its water-holding capacity, but the bacterial cells formed will also make a contribution to the total faecal output. Some effects of various sources of dietary fibre on faecal bulking are illustrated in Fig. 3.3, which contains data for the rat. The points are average values for wet and dry faecal mass, corrected for variations in the food intake of individual animals. The closed (wet mass) and open (dry mass) circles, without error bars, show the almost linear increase in faecal mass that occurs as the cellulose content of the diet is raised. The contribution of wheat bran, sugar beet fibre and guar gum to faecal mass is also shown. All three materials were included in the diet at the 10% level, but of course wheat bran and sugar beet fibre both contain substantially less than 100% dietary fibre. The diagram illustrates the fact that, because of their much greater susceptibility to fermentation, both guar gum and sugar beet fibre provide substantially less faecal mass than the equivalent quantity of cellulose.

Eastwood and Morris (1992) have developed a descriptive equation which attempts to quantify all the complex effects of dietary fibre on faecal bulk:

$$\text{Stool Weight} = W_f(1+H_f) + W_b(1+H_b) + W_m(1+H_m)$$

Where:

W_f = dry weight of fibre after fermentation

W_b = dry weight of bacteria

W_m = dry weight of osmotically active metabolites

H_f = *water-holding capacity of fibre

H_b = *water-holding capacity of bacteria

H_m = *water-holding capacity of metabolites

Apart from the recovery of water, endogenous secretions and energy from food components that have escaped digestion, the major function of

*Water-holding capacity is defined as the weight of water that is resistant to absorption in the colon, per unit dry weight of faecal constituent.

bacterial fermentation in the colon is to regulate the physical and chemical properties of the intraluminal environment. The colonic mucosa is much more susceptible to cancer than that of the small bowel and this may well be because it is exposed to carcinogenic components of faecal material throughout the lifetime of the individual. Fermentation of carbohydrate

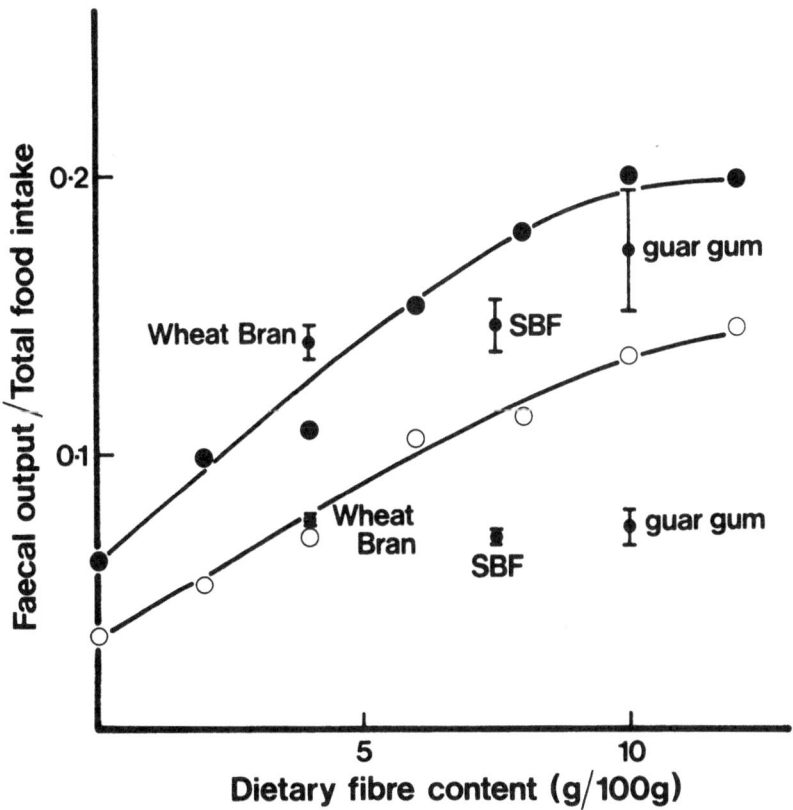

Figure 3.3
Mean values for wet and dry faecal output of rats, corrected for variations in the food intake, plotted against the dietary fibre content of a semisynthetic diet. There was an almost linear increase in dry (O) and wet (●) faecal mass as the cellulose content of the diet was raised. The contribution of wheat bran, sugar beet fibre (SBF) and guar gum to faecal mass is also shown. These materials were included in the diet at the 10% level, but the wheat bran and sugar beet fibre contained only about 45% and 75% dietary fibre respectively. (Reproduced from Johnson et al. [1990] with permission from the British Journal of Nutrition.)

reduces the pH of the colonic contents, and increases the quantity of butyrate available to the mucosal cells. These changes may reduce the production of carcinogenic chemicals and lessen the susceptibility of the colonic mucosal cells to neoplastic change. On the other hand, in experimental animals, volatile fatty acids have been shown to stimulate the rate at which colonic mucosal cells are replicated, and this could have an adverse effect on the induction and fixation of genetic damage. Despite the epidemiological evidence for a protective effect of dietary fibre against colorectal cancer in man, the precise role and mechanisms of action of particular cell wall polysaccharides in the Western diet remain uncertain.

The other products of carbohydrate fermentation are volatile fatty acids, and flatus gas, some of which probably accumulates in the colonic contents in the form of minute bubbles. These components do not contribute to total faecal mass, but they probably a play a major role in bowel function by stimulating colorectal motility, softening the texture of the faeces and increasing their total volume.

Changes in the duration of faecal transit are closely linked to the faecal bulking effect of fibre. Food traverses the oesophagus within a few seconds, but in most individuals the head of a meal takes about 4 hours to reach the colon. Some residual components of a meal may appear in the faeces within about 12 hours after consumption, but the total time needed for all traces of the meal to disappear from the alimentary tract can be several days. Transit times vary considerably, both between populations and between and within individuals. There is little doubt that differences in the type and quantity of dietary fibre consumed are partly responsible for such variation. In the small intestine, complex plant foods that retain the integrity of their cell walls are delayed in transit compared to soluble non-absorbable sugars such as lactulose. In contrast, a high intake of dietary fibre usually leads to a faster transit time through the colon, so that there is an inverse relationship between faecal bulk and the length of time that faecal material is retained in the large bowel. This is probably due to stimulation of colonic motility by a high intraluminal mass.

3.5.3 Colonic Obstruction

Having successfully traversed the small intestine, cell wall polysaccharides might seem unlikely to cause any obstruction to the healthy colon, which after all is adapted to accommodate and propel bulky, semisolid faecal materials. Judging from the literature, this expectation is generally justified. Obstruction of the colon has occasionally been reported, but the few cases that have been described seem to have been due to enormous overconsumption of unprocessed bran. These events can probably be regarded more as clinical curiosities than as indicators of any general risk (*Kang & Dow, 1979*).

FURTHER READING

British Nutrition Foundation. *Complex Carbohydrates in Foods. Report of the British Nutrition Foundation Task Force.* London: Chapman & Hall, 1991.

Burkitt DP, Trowell HC, eds. *Refined Carbohydrate Foods: Some Implications of Dietary Fibre.* London: Academic Press, 1975.

Schweizer TF, Edwards CA, eds. *Dietary Fibre: A Component of Food.* London: Springer Verlag, 1992.

Southgate DAT, Waldron K, Johnson IT, Fenwick GR, eds. *Dietary Fibre: Chemical and Biological Aspects.* Cambridge: Royal Society of Chemistry, 1991.

CHAPTER
—4—

The Antinutritional Effects of Cell Wall Polysaccharides

As we have seen, one of the most consistent effects of increasing the intake of dietary fibre is a rise in the excretion of both wet and dry weight of faeces. This is associated with greater faecal losses of energy, and a consequent reduction in the apparent digestibility of the energy in the diet. ('Apparent digestibility' is defined as intake minus faecal excretion, divided by intake. It may be expressed as a percentage or a proportion.) Although some of the increased faecal material consists of undigested cell wall material, this is often accompanied by nitrogenous matter and lipids so that the apparent digestibilities of both protein and fat are reduced. At the levels of dietary fibre consumption that are typical of the UK, such faecal losses are small but statistically significant. The increases in excreted organic matter also contain bacterial debris and this, to a certain extent, makes the exact interpretation of the faecal losses in terms of dietary intakes somewhat difficult. However, one thing that can be said is that any increase in bacterial mass must have occurred at the expense of the host since it is ultimately derived from food materials that have not been absorbed.

The increased faecal losses of organic matter are associated with an elevated excretion of inorganic substances, especially potassium, phosphorus, magnesium and calcium. Characteristically there is a smaller absolute increase in sodium excretion, although the proportional increase in sodium loss is greater because of the higher faecal water content (*Southgate, 1975*). The increased faecal excretion of inorganic substances results in lower apparent absorptions of these nutrients. ('Apparent absorption' is directly analogous to 'apparent digestibility', a term that is usually restricted to organic constituents.) In general, these effects on faecal losses of both organic and inorganic constituents could be interpreted as an antinutritional effect of dietary fibre or plant cell wall materials because the increased consumption of these constituents has reduced the nutritional value of the diet.

The adverse effect of dietary fibre on the apparent absorption of inorganic nutrients attracted considerable attention when the dietary fibre hypothesis was first proposed because this was seen as a contraindication to the general advice that the hypothesis was propounding (*Southgate, 1987*). Indeed it has frequently been argued that a general recommendation for everyone to increase their intakes of dietary fibre may be inappropriate because those for whom mineral nutrition is critical, such as infants, older children, pregnant women and the elderly, might thereby have their nutritional status compromised.

In this chapter we consider the effects of dietary fibre on nutrient absorption, the possible mechanisms involved, and the significance of the effects of increasing dietary fibre intakes on nutritional status.

——4.1——
CHARACTERISTICS OF DIETS RICH IN DIETARY FIBRE

In examining the effects of dietary fibre on nutrient absorption it is important to reiterate the proposition mentioned earlier in Chapter 1: a diet that is rich in plant cell wall material differs in many other respects from a diet that is poor in these materials (see Table 1.1). In making this statement we are referring to diets composed of foods as eaten by a human population, not to those eaten by experimental subjects. For the purposes of this discussion, a low intake is seen as being of the order of 6-10 g of NSP a day (approximately 10-15 g of TDF), and high intakes would be defined as ranging between 18 and 24 g of NSP or 30 and 40 g of TDF.

One obvious difference in such diets is that the range of foods consumed differs, and these foods bring different types of proteins and lipids into the diet. Many of these plant foods also contain increased concentrations of inorganic constituents which are often present in the foods in a different range of chemical species when compared with a low-fibre diet. The presence of the plant tissues also confers structural features on the distribution and localization of the nutrients. Thus the protein in high-extraction cereals is located in the aleurone layers of the grain, where it is enclosed in thick cell walls. Similarly many of the inorganic constituents are located within the cell walls and some, such as calcium, may be directly combined with the carbohydrates of the wall structures. One particular inorganic nutrient, phosphorus, is often found combined in phytic acid, the hexaphosphate of inositol, where it forms a reserve of inorganic phosphate for germination. Not surprisingly this is particularly true of seeds. Because they have an increased proportion of energy from carbohydrate these diets also have a lower proportion of their energy as fat (which also tends to be less saturated because of the increased proportion of plant oils) and the animal proteins tend to be lower as a proportion of the total protein (*Perisse et al., 1969; Southgate, 1988*).

Thus, in association with a higher intake of plant cell walls we also have a substantial number of qualitative and quantitative differences in the nutrients present. Further, the plant foods bring a range of other biologically active substances into the diet in addition to their vitamins and minerals. These include phenolic materials, ranging from the phenolic acids to complex tannins and lignin (*Gillooly et al., 1983*). This means that, when interpreting an observed increase in the faecal excretion of both organic and inorganic nutrients resulting from an increased consumption of dietary fibre, it is extremely difficult to separate the effects of the diet itself from the effects of the dietary fibre per se. One therefore has to distinguish between the effects of *high-fibre diets* on the one hand and the effects of the *cell wall materials* on the other. In relation to the practical issues of dietary advice to populations, these distinctions are academic but they must nevertheless concern us in interpreting the mechanisms involved.

————4.2————
OBSERVATIONS FROM STUDIES WITH INCREASED INTAKE OF DIETARY FIBRE

Many studies have been reported, starting from the early work of Atwater and Rubner at the beginning of the present century, which demonstrate that increasing the intake of high-extraction cereal foods results in elevated faecal losses of energy, protein and fats (reviewed by *Merrill & Watt, 1955*). These early studies were interpreted as evidence for a lower intrinsic digestibility of the proteins and lipids in these foods. Subsequently many studies have confirmed both the observations and, to a considerable extent, their interpretation. The experimental approach invariably involved the substitution of foods to achieve the higher intakes (see, for example, *Southgate & Durnin, 1970*), which precluded any distinction between the effects of the diet and the dietary fibre. To achieve this the design of the study would need to be such that only the dietary fibre had been changed. Such experiments are not simple to design because of the complexity of the dietary fibre in foods, and the fact that virtually all diets, except very strictly formulated semisynthetic ones, contain some dietary fibre.

Studies using preparations of dietary fibre or plant cell walls have shown that these reduce the apparent absorption of inorganic nutrients in humans but the results obtained by different workers are somewhat inconsistent (*Frølich, 1992*). The major problem is that these preparations are complex mixtures and usually contain substantial concentrations of inorganic nutrients, in addition to proteins and other constituents of the plant including phytates and polyphenolic materials. Other studies have attempted to resolve these difficulties by feeding isolated polysaccharides as 'models' of the components of the plant cell wall. Experiments using isolated pectins, hemicelluloses, cellulose preparations, gums such as guar gum, and mucilages such as ispaghula (a complex branched arabinoxylan), have been conducted with both human subjects and experimental animals (*Prynne & Southgate, 1979*). Some of these materials were already commercially available as food ingredients and were widely used in early studies because they could be fed to human subjects without ethical concerns. Polysaccharides isolated from plant cell wall materials carry concerns about the safety of the reagents used in their isolation, and in many cases the amounts extracted were small so that the experiments had to be restricted to small animals. These studies showed that, even when there were no changes in the proteins or lipids in the diet, the feeding of increased amounts of the isolated polysaccharides resulted in greater faecal losses of nitrogenous material and lipids. Such findings indicate that there is an effect on the digestibility of these organic dietary components which is attributable to the polysaccharide fed.

However, the results for the excretion of inorganic nutrients have been generally less clear-cut and often inconsistent between studies. Most show that isolated polysaccharides do not increase the faecal losses of most inorganic nutrients (*Frølich, 1992; Rossander et al., 1992*). Observations obtained with isolated cellulose are exceptional in that some cellulose preparations appear to increase faecal losses of calcium and magnesium (*Slavin & Marlett, 1980*), and possibly also zinc, although these studies are less well-controlled. It is important to recognize that some of the reported effects of cellulose relate to studies with cellulose preparations that are soluble, and have had acidic groups inserted to enable them to be used as the sodium salts (*Frølich, 1992*). Accordingly, it is difficult to extrapolate these effects to cellulose as it occurs in the plant cell wall. The general conclusion from most of this work is therefore that isolated neutral polysaccharides do not have adverse effects on mineral absorption.

Some reports of effects on vitamin absorption have been reported but, again, these usually refer to diets where the food mixture has been altered and are therefore difficult to interpret strictly in terms of a effect of dietary fibre.

———4.3———
POSSIBLE MECHANISMS FOR THE EFFECTS ON DIGESTION OF NUTRIENTS

In considering the mechanisms for the effects of dietary fibre on the digestion of nutrients it is important to focus on events in the small intestine, rather than to rely on apparent digestibility values obtained from faecal analysis. Interpretation of faecal excretion in terms of unabsorbed dietary components is very problematic, especially with the organic components, because of the profound changes, both quantitative and qualitative, that the activities of the large intestinal microflora produce in these components during caecal fermentation (*Southgate, 1989*). Furthermore the large amounts of bacterial debris in faeces also confounds the interpretation (*Stephen & Cummings, 1980*), as it does with nutrients such as the B-vitamins which may be synthesized by the microflora. Finally, it must be recognized that faecal material contains components of the diet that have been concentrated during passage. Thus pigments, artificial colours, mineral oil and a range of heat-induced, indigestible artefacts produced by cooking are also present at measurable concentrations, whereas in the diet their concentrations would be regarded as insignificant (*Southgate, 1973*). Human faecal excretion is often only 3–5% of the dry matter taken in as food so, clearly, substantial concentration has taken place.

4.3.1 Effects of the Structure of the Diet

A high-fibre diet is typically bulky with a relatively low density. This has effects on gastric activity, since for a given amount of food the stomach will be filled earlier, so that gastric emptying and possibly satiety may be modified. In animals, bulk is known to have depressing effects on voluntary food consumption, but in humans the effects are less well-documented. Anecdotal evidence from the use of bulking polysaccharides such as methylcellulose in 'slimming' preparations suggests that there is some effect on voluntary food intake over a short period of time but this is not clearly established. In young children the bulk of the diet may limit food intake, and where the nutrient density of the diet (that is the kcal or kJ per g of diet) is low, as occurs in some rural African diets, this can result in the child failing to fulfil its energy needs (*Rutishauser & Whitehead, 1972*). It is difficult, however, to envisage effects on gastric emptying as having significant effects on small intestinal digestion overall, because of the very high absorptive capacity of the human intestinal tract.

4.3.2 The Effects of Cell Wall Structures

The ability of the physical structure of foods containing plant cell walls to confer physical properties on the contents of the intestinal tract, and to compartmentalize the component nutrients of foods, was described in the last chapter. Thus the nutrients may be contained within cellular structures in which the cell walls themselves act as barriers to diffusion from the cell, and possibly to the diffusion of digestive secretions into the cells. This type of mechanism probably accounts for the fact that diets rich in wholegrain cereals lead to faecal energy losses that are higher than with diets containing similar amounts of fruit or vegetable fibre (*Livesey, 1992*).

As the plant cell wall material moves through the intestine, the removal of digestible components strips the cell wall surfaces, and the mixing of the gut facilitates the hydration, solution and dispersion of soluble components into the gut contents. The surface areas of cell walls exposed during digestion are very extensive and, while little is known of their surface properties, it is probable that these surfaces are capable of adsorbing inorganic ions and other molecules.

The soluble components of the cell wall polysaccharides include several types of NCP that produce viscous solutions or gels. While the conditions for the formation of gels are unlikely to be met in the intestine, the main effects will be on viscosity. Many of the soluble polysaccharides contain free carboxyl groups and these will have become dissociated in the stomach and so be present as the free carboxyl groups in the small intestine. They will therefore be capable of combining with divalent ions. Furthermore the physical effects of the soluble polysaccharides include a weak surface-active property so that effects on micellar formation are possible, with as yet poorly understood consequences for fat absorption.

———4.4———
EFFECTS ON ORGANIC NUTRIENTS

4.4.1 Proteins

The reduced apparent digestibility of protein in diets rich in plant cell wall materials appears to be due to a combination of effects. First, some of the plant proteins are integral parts of the plant cell wall. There is evidence suggesting that these proteins are intrinsically less digestible than the more soluble cytoplasmic or storage proteins because they possess some analogous structural features with the extracellular proteins of animal tissues (*Saunders & Betschart, 1980*). All simulated proteolytic digestions of plant material leave some residual unhydrolysed protein. Second, as mentioned before, storage proteins are located within cells with thickened walls, especially those of cereals and seed legumes. In raw foods these walls are resistant to physical disintegration and the proteins only become significantly digestible if the tissues are heated in moist conditions which lead to the disruption of the intercellular structures.

There is also some evidence from animal studies that the consumption of diets rich in plant cell wall material can lead to increased losses of endogenous proteins from mucosal tissues, due to mechanical damage to the intestinal wall. However, the importance of this type of effect in humans consuming relatively softened cell wall structures is difficult to assess.

Finally, many plant foods contain proteins such as lectins and enzyme inhibitors which, in raw foods, would reduce protein digestibility. Most of these substances are denatured by heat so the effects are only important when raw or inadequately cooked foods are consumed. The properties and antinutritional effects of such substances are discussed in greater detail in Chapter 6.

4.4.2 Fats

The interpretation of the reduced apparent digestibilities of fats observed in many studies is complicated by the fact that in most cases only total lipids have been measured. The problem of distinguishing between the effects of dietary fibre and other characteristics of the diet is encountered again because increasing the intake of plant foods also leads to a greater intake of complex lipids such as cutins and waxes, together with plant sterols. All of these compounds contribute to indigestible lipid in the faeces. It is probable that in many studies the lipids in these diets are intrinsically less digestible. Nevertheless, some isolated polysaccharides such as pectin, guar gum and ispaghula do increase the faecal excretion of simple lipids from purified diets, suggesting that there are independent effects on lipid absorption. The fact that all these polysaccharides have physical effects on the intestinal contents implies that the effects on absorption may be due to interference with the stability or diffusion of mixed micelles in the intestinal contents.

4.4.3 Vitamins

There are relatively few reports of the effects of dietary fibre on vitamin absorption, especially of the water-soluble vitamins. Some observations on the binding of folates to polysaccharides have been reported but the significance of these effects is difficult to assess. The consumption of increased amounts of plant foods, and especially of vegetables, would lead to increased intakes of folates so that the nutritional significance of any binding effects would almost certainly be negligible.

Recent interests in the carotenoid components of the diet have produced some evidence that the absorption of carotenoids from plant foods is greatly dependent on the physical state of the plant tissue. This suggests that when the cellular structures are retained absorption is greatly reduced. Again, the explanation may be that the physical structure of the cell wall acts as a barrier and prevents the carotenoids from dispersing and entering the mixed micelles. The low proportions of fats commonly associated with these diets may also contribute to the poor absorption.

———4.5———
EFFECTS OF DIETARY FIBRE ON ABSORPTION OF INORGANIC NUTRIENTS

As mentioned earlier, most attention has been focussed on the effects of dietary fibre on the absorption of inorganic nutrients, and especially of calcium, iron and zinc. The remainder of this chapter is concerned with assessing the evidence for adverse nutritional effects of this kind.

4.5.1 Physical Chemical Studies of Isolated Polysaccharides

The complexity of the dietary fibre mixture, and the difficulties of controlling conditions in the small intestine *in vivo* or *in vitro*, have led many workers to investigate the physical properties of isolated polysaccharides in an attempt to establish the nature of the effects of dietary fibre on nutrient absorption. The properties of uronans such as pectin and the alginates in regard to the reactions with divalent cations have been studied extensively. The carboxyl groups react with cations at pHs similar to those found in the small intestine and binding appears to involve intermolecular chelation to form strong gels. There is some evidence that the hydroxyl groups are also involved in the binding that is observed with methoxylated pectins. The strength and other properties of the gels depend upon the binding constants of the cations. Of the major inorganic nutrients, calcium is bound more strongly than copper, zinc and iron, with magnesium being relatively weakly bound. In *in vitro* binding studies, neutral polysaccharides show very weak or zero binding, although it is possible to envisage that the hydroxyl groups may show a weak tendency to dissociate or form hydrogen bonds.

In vitro binding of calcium has been observed at physiological pHs with cell wall preparations from a range of fruits and vegetables, and was highly correlated with the uronic acid content of the preparations

(*James et al., 1978*). The pH-dependence of the binding was also consistent with the uronic acids being involved. Studies with some neutral polysaccharides show binding effects at higher pHs than found physiologically which are difficult to interpret. This is also true for studies of cellulose preparations that show evidence of binding of calcium, iron and zinc. It is possible that the binding is due to adsorption to the surfaces of these fibres, the binding capacity of which may have been modified during extraction.

4.5.2 Technical Limitations of In Vitro Studies

In vitro studies of the physical properties of isolated polysaccharide 'models', and of isolated fibre preparations, are extremely attractive because they can be carried out relatively rapidly under carefully controlled conditions. They can therefore be used in the development and measurement of physicochemical constants for binding or cation exchange capacity. Such experiments are essential for mechanistic investigations. In the present context the aim is to develop predictive models for the behaviour and effects on mineral nutrition of dietary fibre and its components. It is therefore essential to consider the limitations and advantages of *in vitro* techniques in detail (*Southgate, 1989*).

Preparation of the material under investigation

Although one could argue that isolated polysaccharides do not undergo preparation, all such polysaccharides have undergone some kind of physical or chemical treatment. Thus pectins have been extracted under acid conditions which effectively depolymerizes the native molecules and dissociates all the associated cations. The binding properties will thus be profoundly influenced by the provenance of the sample. Similarly most of the algal polysaccharides have been subjected to acid conditions during extraction. Materials such as guar, ispaghula and the exudate gums may have had only comparatively mild physical treatments such as sieving or washing. The situation is more complex in the case of materials isolated from the plant cell wall because many fractions, for example 'hemicellulose' preparations, are only extractable after alkaline treatment, and this may have produced some beta-elimination reactions, introducing functional groups not normally present. Most cellulose preparations derived from woody tissues will have been treated with strong oxidizing agents to remove lignin, and these are known to introduce carboxyl groups in the disordered regions of the cellulose fibres, thus altering their cation-exchange capabilities. There are many examples of binding which almost certainly represent artefactual effects due to the preparation of the materials being studied (*Frølich et al., 1984*).

Co-precipitation effects

These can be of two types, the first of which relates to the changes in the material being studied. For example, many polysaccharides are isolated by ethanolic precipitation at around 80% v/v. This can alter the physical characteristics of the polysaccharide molecule, and also lead to co-precipitation of proteins which modify the properties of the polysaccharide. The second type of effect occurs when pH adjustments are made when one is studying the binding at different pHs. Taking a polysaccharide through a cycle of pHs may co-precipitate the component whose binding is being studied and the component may only slowly redissolve later in the experiment. This effect occurred during preliminary studies of bile salt binding to fibre preparations, leading initially to erroneous identification of the active binding component. The remedy for these types of effect lies in the use of techniques such as dialysis to isolate polysaccharides, and the avoidance of dehydrating conditions such as strong ethanolic solutions. In all polysaccharide studies, extreme pH values should be avoided, and the pH adjustments made before adding the component whose binding is being investigated.

Measurement of binding

Most *in vitro* systems attempt to simulate the conditions in the intestine with respect to pH and ionic strengths, but usually utilize arbitrary ranges for the concentrations of both the polysaccharide and the nutrient whose binding is being studied. There is widespread use of dialysis to assess the proportion of nutrient that is unbound (*Miller et al., 1981*). This may be done under equilibrium conditions after some time period, chosen experimentally, where diffusion across the membrane reaches a plateau. Many authors consider that this does not adequately simulate physiological conditions where a nutrient is being progressively removed from the intestinal contents. If this argument is accepted it follows that binding should be assessed against a simulation of the continual gradient that is produced as a nutrient is absorbed. Continuous dialysis methods have been developed recently and these show that binding is slightly lower using continuous techniques (*Wolthers, 1992*). These techniques have also been used to measure binding constants for dietary fibre preparations and a range of inorganic nutrients. By using a range of different fibre preparations it is possible to derive regression equations relating the binding to the presence of specific monosaccharide components of the dietary fibre.

Simulation of physiological conditions

Dealing with the issue of continuous removal of nutrients from the intestinal lumen is only one of the difficulties encountered in modelling physiological factors *in vitro*. The other effects, which concern the simulation of mucosal transport, are more problematic. Many nutrients are absorbed actively, that is against a concentration gradient, by specific transport mechanisms located at the luminal poles of the mucosal cells. Clearly these can only be simulated using a physiological preparation of intestine. The effect of the dietary fibre on nutrient absorption will be a function of the ratio between the binding constants for the polysaccharide and the binding constant of the transport site. In addition, interactions occur between nutrients competing for transport sites, and between nutrients and other components of the diet. For example, proteins and surface-active compounds such as saponins alter transport rates and will therefore tend to confound any estimate of the effects of dietary fibre on nutrient absorption.

The absorption of many micronutrients is regulated by physiological mechanisms that operate through biological feedback systems. This means that no model for the effects of dietary fibre on nutrient absorption can be described in terms of diffusion or binding constants alone. Thus the extent to which *in vitro* measurements of binding can be interpreted in terms of effects on nutrient absorption is limited. The results from *in vitro* studies should always be considered alongside comparable studies *in vivo*, and the value of an *in vitro* assessment must be judged in terms of how well it predicts effects on nutrient absorption *in vivo*.

-----4.6-----
EVIDENCE FROM STUDIES USING ILEOSTOMISTS

Patients who have had their large intestine resected because of colonic disease provide a 'model' for investigating the effects of dietary fibre on nutrient absorption in the small intestine. These patients have the small intestine brought to a stoma on the abdominal wall and the effluent from the small intestine is collected in a bag. The operation is of course a radical one that imposes considerable stress on the individual. Great care and attention to ethical issues is required in the study of these patients because they become very acutely aware of the effects of dietary changes on the behaviour of their small intestine. The 'model' is also not a perfect one because some bacterial colonization of the lower small intestine is difficult to prevent, and because the constraints on intestinal flow produced by the ileocaecal valve in the intact condition have been removed.

Despite their limitations, experiments with ileostomists have provided some valuable insights into the effects of dietary fibre preparations on mineral absorption. These studies show that neutral polysaccharides do not increase the proportion of inorganic nutrients reaching the end of the small intestine, but that acidic polysaccharides such as pectin do reduce the intestinal absorption of iron. Preparations that are rich in phytates have the strongest effects in reducing the absorption and these effects are largely abolished when the phytates are removed enzymatically (*Rossander et al., 1992*)

———4.7———
NUTRITIONAL SIGNIFICANCE OF EFFECTS OF DIETARY FIBRE ON NUTRIENT ABSORPTION

A number of observational studies made on population groups that habitually consume high-fibre intakes have been reported. These groups were in the main vegetarian ones and where energy intakes were satisfactory there was no evidence of depressed mineral status. No doubt this was in part due to the fact that these diets usually had higher inorganic nutrient densities, so that despite the lower percentage apparent absorptions the net retention of inorganic nutrients was positive. Studies with vegetarian women have shown that, when the vegetarian diet is being consumed as part of a weight-control regimen, depressed iron status can be seen. This has also been observed in Scandinavian men who had very high intakes of dietary fibre as a result of their high levels of energy expenditure. (This observation is linked to the Scandinavian formulation of dietary recommendations on an energy basis.) In all these cases the overall effects of high-fibre diets are being observed, rather than effects of dietary fibre per se, and all these high-fibre intakes were associated with higher levels of phytates and polyphenolic materials.

Studies with high intakes of pectin show no effects on faecal calcium excretion or calcium status. This leads to the question of the apparent discrepancy between the well-established effects of acidic polysaccharides in binding divalent nutrients and the absence of significant effects *in vivo* when these polysaccharides are fed at substantial levels. In part this is due to the difficulties of simulating intestinal digestion and absorption *in vitro* discussed earlier. Furthermore most studies of *in vitro* binding have not included the simulation of the caecal fermentation stage. In the pectin study mentioned, no pectin could be detected in the faecal matter, showing that fermentation had been complete, and any bound constituents would have been released into the large bowel. Although mineral absorption rates in the large bowel are low, the residence times at this site are high and significant recovery of mineral nutrients probably occurs.

———4.8———
SUMMARY

Consumption of some types of dietary fibre reduces the apparent digestibility of energy and organic nutrients, but these effects will be negligible for most Western consumers. The apparent absorption of mineral nutrients is also reduced by some high-fibre diets. Although many of the polysaccharide components of plant cell walls, especially those with acidic functional groups, bind divalent inorganic nutrients *in vitro*, there is no convincing evidence that the increased consumption of these polysaccharides leads to reduced absorption of inorganic nutrients. One must therefore reject the hypothesis that increased intakes of dietary fibre exert antinutritional effects in respect of inorganic nutrients. The reductions in the apparent absorption of inorganic nutrients observed when diets rich in high-extraction cereal foods are consumed appear to be due almost entirely to the effects of the phytates associated with the cereal foods, and probably to polyphenolic compounds also associated with these diets. Thus, when making dietary recommendations to increase the intake of dietary fibre to groups of the population where mineral status is critical, the focus should be on drawing the dietary fibre intake from sources that are low in phytate, and on maintaining adequate intakes of inorganic nutrients; if this is done there are no significant concerns about effects on mineral status (*Southgate, 1987; Stanstead et al., 1979; Gordon, 1994*).

FURTHER READING

James WPT. Dietary fiber and mineral absorption. In: *Medical Aspects of Dietary Fiber*. Spiller GA, McPherson K, eds. New York: Plenum Medical Book Co., 1980, pp 239–59.

Livesey G. The energy values of dietary fibre and sugar alcohols for man. *Nutr Res Rev.* 1992; 5: 61–84

Southgate DAT. Minerals, trace elements, and potential hazards. *Am J Clin Nutr* 1987; 45: 1256–66.

Southgate D, Johnson IT, Fenwick GR, eds. *Nutrient Availability: Chemical and Biological Aspects*. Cambridge: Royal Society of Chemistry, 1989.

CHAPTER

—5—

Effects of Dietary Fibre on Mucosal Cell Proliferation

The surface of the human small intestinal mucosa is covered by an array of finger-like or leaf-like processes, the villi. Each villus consists of an inner core of mesenchymal cells, blood and lymph vessels, nerves and connective tissue, and an outer surface layer or sheet of columnar epithelial cells. The epithelium contains both absorptive cells and mucus-secreting goblet cells. Beneath the villi are blind, glandular crypts, which open into the intestinal lumen at the bases of the villi. As early as 1892 the Italian pathologist Bizzozero had recognized that the mucosal surface was a dynamic tissue, containing transient elements or *elementi labili*, and that the whole structure was constantly in a state of renewal. He was the first to suggest that cells shed into the lumen from the tips of the villi were replaced by new cells migrating outwards from the crypts. This conjecture was confirmed with the advent of modern techniques such as autoradiography, which is used to detect and localize radioactively la-belled DNA precursors within cells and tissues.

Under low-power microscopy the mucosal surfaces of the large intestine appear strikingly different from those of the jejunum and ileum. Villi are entirely absent and, apart from relatively inconspicuous surface ridges and a regular array of crypt orifices, the surface of the colon is smooth and featureless. The lack of villi in the colon reflects the slow rates of solute and fluid transport that occur there, and perhaps also the need to withstand the stresses associated with the passage of abrasive faecal material. Nevertheless the fundamental organization of the mucosal surfaces, and the processes of epithelial replication, are similar in the small and large intestines.

The origin of intestinal epithelial cells is a small population of relatively slowly dividing stem cells near the base of each crypt. This population gives rise to 'amplification-division' cells which proliferate rapidly during their migration away from the basal region. In normal mucosa, the cells become differentiated beyond the stage at which further replication is possible by the time they reach the upper third of the crypt. In the small intestine they continue to mature and express carrier and digestive enzyme activity as they leave the crypt orifice and ascend the villus column. The average cell cycle time is approximately 11.5 hours in normal tissue, and the lifespan of a differentiating human mucosal cell is about 3.5 days. It has been estimated that the total production of mucosal cells for the entire human small intestine amounts to about 35 million cells per minute, equivalent to a cell mass of about 250 g per day. This intense activity makes the alimentary tract the major site of protein synthesis in adult humans but most of the cellular constituents are simply diluted by dietary components and efficiently re-absorbed.

Despite the very high rates of cellular proliferation that take place in the gastrointestinal tissues, the morphological characteristics of the mucosal surfaces remain remarkably constant over time. This means that under normal circumstances cellular production and loss are precisely balanced. Clearly a high degree of physiological control is being exerted, but the mucosa can also respond adaptively to physiological and environmental stimuli. The mechanisms underlying these homeostatic and adaptive processes are incompletely understood, and their complete explication remains a major challenge. Much of the work that has been done has been carried out using experimental animals, but the study of human intestinal adaptation following surgical resection for the treatment of ischaemia, inflammatory disease or morbid obesity has also provided a great deal of information.

The small intestine is highly sensitive to changes in the quantity and composition of nutrients. The most extreme challenge is complete starvation, which gives rise to large reductions in tissue weight, in the dimensions of the crypts and the villi, and the size of the proliferating compartment. These morphological changes are associated with a prolongation of the cell cycle and a reduction in the rate of migration. The importance of intraluminal nutrients as direct stimuli for cellular replication is demonstrated by the fact that the effects of food withdrawal are not prevented by intravenous nutrition.

Surgical removal of the proximal small intestine removes the principal site of nutrient absorption and exposes the distal mucosa to unusually high concentrations of nutrients, and hence to an increase in the 'workload' of absorption. This provides a powerful stimulus for adaptation in the remnant. One of the first events after surgery is a small reduction in the S phase of the cell cycle in the proliferating crypt cell compartment at sites both proximal and distal to the site of resection. Within a few days there is a permanent increase in both total crypt cell population and the size of the proliferating compartment, which is directly proportional to the total length of the small bowel that has been resected. In the normal small bowel there is a gradient of villous height and cellularity such that the duodenal and jejunal villi are taller and more richly vascularized that those of the ileum. After resection of the proximal small bowel, the ileum takes on many of the morphological and functional characteristics of the missing tissue. In both animals and humans these changes in cellular replication and morphology are accompanied by adaptive changes in function. Jejunal resection leads to increased segmental rates of absorption of electrolytes and organic nutrients. These increases tend to counterbalance the diminished absorptive capacity, so that eventually much of the original functional capacity of the intestine is recovered.

The secretions of the pancreas and biliary tract enter the duodenum during the digestive process. They are rich in bile acids, proteins and lipids of endogenous origin, some of which have been shown to be trophic to the mucosa. This has led some to suggest that it is the modulation of pancreatic and biliary secretion produced by changes in food intake which leads to adaptive changes in the mucosa, rather than the direct effects of the nutrients themselves. Secondary bile acids produced by bacterial metabolism of primary bile acids reaching the large bowel may be damaging to the colonic mucosa and may stimulate proliferation to replace lost cells. Clearly these endogenous secretions play some role in the control of small intestinal growth, but they are only one component of a complex system.

Strong evidence that one or more hormonal factors are involved in the control of intestinal adaptation comes from parabiotic studies in which the circulation of a treated animal is 'crossed' with that of an untreated individual or 'parabiont'. This type of experiment has been used to show that intestinal resection in the treated animal induces adaptive changes in the recipient. Similarly, within a single individual, exclusion of a length of small bowel from the normal nutrient flow leads to hypoplasia, but this effect can be prevented by substantial resection of the remaining functionally intact intestine. These experiments strongly support the possibility that some bloodborne factor or trophic hormone is involved in small intestinal adaptation.

Finally the metabolic activities of the resident intestinal microflora appear to be important in the maintenance of normal mucosal cell replication. In ruminants the products of fermentation are known to stimulate crypt cell proliferation in the ruminal mucosa. A number of studies with rodents suggest that the same is true of the colonic mucosa in monogastric mammals. Germ-free animals have a low rate of mucosal cell proliferation in the small bowel, and this has been attributed to the absence of a somewhat ill-defined state of 'physiological inflammation'. Some workers have emphasized the importance of acidification by fermentative microorganisms as a stimulant for cell proliferation in the rat colon, and others suggest that short-chain fatty acids stimulate mucosal cell proliferation directly and should be regarded as 'enterotrophins'. Moreover it has been reported that the introduction of short-chain fatty acids into the colon leads to increased rates of mucosal cell replication in the small bowel, and that this is dependent upon the maintenance of an intact neural network.

In this chapter we will describe the effects of NSP on intestinal mucosal cell proliferation in some detail. The significance of these effects will be described in relation to the maintenance of normal intestinal structure, and the possible implications for human health will be considered.

———5.1———
EFFECTS OF NON-STARCH POLYSACCHARIDES ON NORMAL MUCOSAL CELL REPLICATION

The proposed protective effect of dietary fibre against colorectal cancer has prompted interest in the relationship between fibre intake and mucosal cell proliferation in the large intestine. Research has also focussed on the choice of purified NSP suitable for inclusion in clinical feeds, to prevent mucosal atrophy in tube-fed patients, and to stimulate mucosal healing after intestinal surgery. At the same time there has been an undercurrent of interest in the origin and significance of the subtle morphological changes to the intestinal mucosa, observed under scanning electron microscopy, in rats fed different forms of dietary fibre (*Cassidy et al., 1981*).

Although the one characteristic shared by all NSP is their resistance to digestive enzymes, these substances are by no means inert in the gut lumen. Truly inert dietary bulk has very little effect on mucosal growth. For example, incorporation of finely powdered kaolin into semisynthetic or elemental rat diets at levels as high as 80% by weight has no effect on the proliferation of mucosal epithelial cells in the small or the large bowel, although there is some hypertrophy of the muscle layers. In contrast, the effects of NSP are far more complex, but they vary strikingly from one group of substances to another. It is often suggested that dietary fibre may increase cell proliferation or modify morphology via mechanical damage to the intestinal mucosa. This seems unlikely to be true, however, because coarse insoluble substances like wheat bran have less effect than soluble polysaccharide gums.

The interpretation of the research literature on this topic is hampered by the variety of diets, feeding regimes and experimental end-points which have been used by investigators. In this section the effects of the various classes of dietary fibre will be considered separately, and some attempt will be made to identify general mechanisms of action.

5.1.1 Purified Cellulose

Although cellulose is a major component of the plant cell wall, most of the work on cellulose as a component of dietary fibre has been carried out using purified material. One of the most commonly used types is Solka-Floc® (Johnsen Jorgensen & Wettre Ltd, London), which is an insoluble particulate material derived from wood. The modified cellulose gums will be discussed in a later section.

Purified wood cellulose has proved to be a rather inert material in the gut. It is highly resistant to fermentation when exposed to cultured faecal microorganisms *in vitro* and, when it is fed to monogastric animals as a component of a semisynthetic diet, most of it is recovered in the faeces.

At concentrations up to about 10% by weight, there is an almost linear relationship between dietary cellulose and faecal mass in the rat (Fig. 3.3). A number of research groups have described the effects of purified cellulose on mucosal cell proliferation in the small and large bowel of the rat. In general Solka-Floc® has been found to exert no stimulus to crypt cell production rate at either site (*Johnson et al., 1984*). A comparison of cell proliferation rates at various sites in the alimentary tract of rats given a fibre-free diet or a diet enriched with this type of cellulose is shown in Fig. 5.1. However, purified cellulose does appear to have some ability to prevent the loss of proliferative activity which occurs when very simple or 'elemental' diets are given. For example, Goodlad and Wright (*1983*) reported that the addition of Solka-Floc® (Grade BW-100) to an elemental diet (Flexical®; Mead Johnson Ltd) prevented the reduction in cell division and crypt length seen in the colon when the unsupplemented elemental diet was fed to rats. It would appear therefore that, in relation to the intestinal mucosa, insoluble cellulose is amongst the least biologically active forms of dietary fibre. However, as in many other areas of research on dietary fibre, generalizations are hazardous. Dirks and Freeman (*1987*) have reported that cellulose in the form of Avicel® (FMC Corporation, Philadelphia) increases cell proliferation and crypt length in both the small and the large bowel of the rat. Such contrasting results with seemingly very similar materials probably reflect differences in their physical properties or susceptibility to microbial fermentation which can provide clues to the mechanisms underlying the control of cell proliferation by intraluminal substances.

5.1.2. Cereal Brans

Cereal brans are much more complex materials than the purified celluloses discussed above. They contain lignified insoluble cell wall polysaccharides which strongly resist fermentation by the colonic microflora, as well as varying amounts of soluble cell wall polysaccharides and starch. Unlike Solka-Floc ®, which is virtually 100% dietary fibre, most samples of wheat bran contain only 40–45% dietary fibre. Wheat bran has been widely investigated for its effects on mucosal cell proliferation because it is one of the most common and palatable sources of fibre available for incorporation into human diets. Oat bran has also been studied in some detail because of its increasing popularity as a source of soluble dietary fibre.

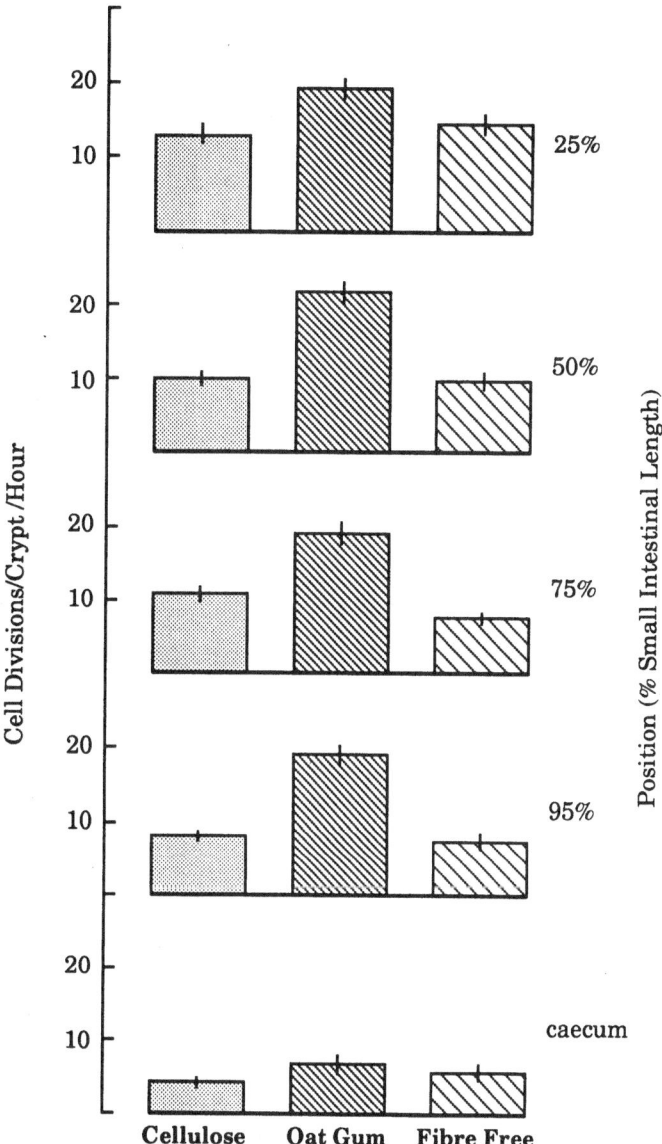

Figure 5.1
Crypt cell production rates at 25%, 50% 75% and 95% of the total small intestinal length, and in the caecum of rats fed a fibre-free diet, or diets containing insoluble cellulose or oat beta-glucan. Cellulose had no significant effect on mitosis but the rate was significantly higher in the animals fed oat gum compared to the control animals at every location.

A number of studies with wheat bran have been carried out using the rat as an experimental model, and most have reported an increase in proliferative activity in the distal colon, but less effect in the proximal colon (*Jacobs & White, 1983*). The small intestine shows little or no proliferative response to wheat bran. In a recent, carefully conducted study, a complex relationship between the dietary intake of wheat bran and colonic mucosal proliferation has been reported. A diet containing 5% wheat bran slowed colonic mucosal cell proliferation compared to a fibre-free diet, but the addition of 10 and 20% wheat bran was associated with a progressive increase (*Boffa et al., 1992*). There is no obvious explanation for this relationship. It is often proposed that the stimulation of mucosal cell turnover by dietary fibre is due to the production of short-chain fatty acids, principally butyrate, by fermentation of NSP. However, there was no positive correlation between butyrate levels and colonic cell production in the Boffa et al. study.

Oat bran, which contains a relatively high proportion of soluble dietary fibre in the form of beta-glucan, has been reported to stimulate cell proliferation in the proximal colon of the rat, though without causing any increase in mucosal tissue mass (*Jacobs & Lupton, 1984*). This difference in the anatomical distribution of proliferative activity probably reflects differences in the fermentability of the constituent NSP of the two types of bran. However, as we shall see in the next section, purified oat gum gives rise to yet another different pattern of mucosal hyperproliferation. Clearly there are a number of different mechanisms whereby NSP modify the pattern of crypt cell replication in the alimentary tract, and their influence varies markedly depending on the source and quantity of fibre in the diet.

5.1.3 Soluble Non-Starch Polysaccharides

As discussed in Chapter 3, interest in soluble forms of dietary fibre was stimulated by the studies of Jenkins and his co-workers on the hypoglycaemic effects of pectin, guar gum and other isolated NSP (*Jenkins et al., 1978*). These highly viscous materials were usually administered to human subjects in liquid test meals containing glucose. However, for studies with experimental animals they have be successfully incorporated into powdered semisynthetic diets and used in long-term feeding experiments with a view to studying intestinal adaptation. The main interest in these polysaccharides arose from their ability to modify nutrient absorption and this has naturally focussed attention on adaptive changes to the small intestinal mucosa.

Guar gum, pectin and isolated oat beta-glucan, fed at a concentration of 5% or more by weight, all stimulate mucosal cell proliferation throughout the gastrointestinal tract of the rat. The same is true of modified cellulose gums such as methylcellulose, Na-carboxymethylcellulose and hydroxypropylmethylcellulose. The increased rate of crypt cell production is often accompanied by minor changes in mucosal morphology, including an increased crypt length, increased villous height and a broadening of the crypt base, which has a characteristic leaf-like shape in the rat. There are also functional modifications to the mucosal epithelium associated with the changes in epithelial cell kinetics, including a reduction in monosaccharide carrier activity and changes in mucosal disaccharidase activity (*Johnson et al., 1984*). Addition of pectin to an elemental diet has been reported to improve significantly ileal and colonic adaptation to massive small bowel resection in the rat (*Koruda et al., 1986*).

------5.2------
MECHANISM OF ACTION

It should now be clear that many types of dietary fibre tend to stimulate the proliferation of intestinal mucosal cells in experimental animals, but the magnitude of the effect varies considerably from one type of polysaccharide to another. It is widely assumed that fermentation of NSP by the colonic microflora plays a major role in the modulation of intestinal cell turnover. This hypothesis seems highly plausible for a number of reasons. Short-chain fatty acids are the major end-product of carbohydrate fermentation both in ruminants and in monogastric mammals. They are present in high concentrations in the rumen where they are known to stimulate the growth of the mucosa. Moreover, it has been demonstrated that short-chain fatty acids are utilized as an energy source by colonic mucosal cells of monogastric mammals, including man. Prolonged lack of fermentable carbohydrate due to malnutrition is thought to lead to mucosal atrophy and loss of colonic function.

Production of short-chain fatty acids leads to a reduction in the pH of the luminal contents. Lupton et al. (*1985*) manipulated the luminal pH in the colon of the rat by dietary means and observed a strong positive relationship between luminal acidity and the proportion of mucosal crypt cells undergoing DNA synthesis. The authors advanced two plausible hypotheses to account for this. One suggestion was that extracellular pH exerted a direct stimulus to cell division by acidifying the cell interior. Alternatively, they proposed that the effect of luminal acidification might be mediated via an indirect effect on bile acid or eicosanoid metabolism. A reduction in the pH of the colonic luminal contents, and an increase in mucosal cell proliferation, are consistently observed in laboratory animals fed fermentable forms of dietary fibre, but such associations, however statistically significant they may be, do not prove the existence of a causal relationship.

This point is emphasized by the work of Sakata (1987), who demonstrated a stimulation of cell proliferation by direct instillation of short-chain fatty acids into the distal ileum of normal and germ-free rats. The effect was independent of the presence of the colonic microflora, and independent of luminal pH. Moreover, there was a dose-dependent relationship between short-chain fatty acid concentration and crypt cell production rate, and the effect was observed in the jejunum, as well as in the distal intestine, close to the site of infusion. Sakata concluded that short-chain fatty acids, and butyrate in particular, should be regarded as intraluminal growth factors for the gut, and that their production from fermentable polysaccharides such as pectin and guar gum could provide a full explanation for the trophic effects of these forms of dietary fibre in the gut. This view was supported to a large extent by the findings of Goodlad et al. (1989) who showed that starved animals showed a marked increase in colonic and small intestinal mucosal cell proliferation when refed with an elemental diet supplemented with fermentable polysaccharides, but the effect was not observed in germ-free rats.

Although the 'fermentation model' for stimulation of intestinal cell proliferation has become widely accepted there is good evidence to show that it does not provide a complete explanation for the trophic effects of fibre. The previously mentioned studies were carried out using laboratory rodents either previously starved, or consuming a fibre-free elemental diet. The animals were then 'challenged' with a test diet containing fibre, so that each, in effect, acted as its own control. In other experimental models the control animals are simply fed a basal diet either free of fibre, or supplemented with some material against which the 'treatment' polysaccharide is to be compared. Under these circumstances animals fed fermentable polysaccharides such as guar gum, pectin, or oat beta-glucan maintain high rates of cell proliferation compared to control animals fed fibre-free or cellulose-enriched control diets. However, under similar conditions, modified cellulose food gums such as Nacarboxymethyl-cellulose and hydroxypropylmethylcellulose also stimulate high rates of mucosal cell proliferation (*Johnson & Gee, 1986*). These polysaccharides are almost entirely resistant to fermentation, and they tend to cause a slightly alkaline pH in the colonic lumen of the rat (*Wyatt et al., 1988*). Moreover, although certain forms of fermentable fibre do not stimulate mucosal cell proliferation in the absence of an intact colonic flora, this is not true of guar gum, which has been shown to cause an increase in the rate of cell turnover in the jejunal and colonic mucosa of germ-free mice (*Pell et al., 1993*).

The distribution of mitotic activity in laboratory animals fed guar gum, modified cellulose gums, or oat beta-glucan seems to be incompatible with a local direct effect of acidity or short chain fatty acids. This is illustrated in Fig. 5.1, which provides a comparison of crypt cell production rates at several sites in the alimentary tract of rats fed diets containing either insoluble cellulose or oat beta-glucan. The rate of cell proliferation is significantly higher in the animals fed oat gum compared to the control animals at every location. It is extremely unlikely that any significant fermentation of oat gum occurs in the proximal jejunum. If fermentation is the principal stimulus it must act via some intermediate endocrine or neural pathway. Sakata and his co-workers recognized this phenomenon and demonstrated that the direct instillation of short-chain fatty acids into the colon led to a small but significant increase in the rate of crypt cell mitosis in areas of the gut remote from stimulus, including the small bowel and parts of the stomach (*Sakata & Yajima, 1984*). This experiment provided clear evidence to suggest the existence of some kind of physiological signal pathway linking events in the colonic lumen to the rest of the alimentary tract. One obvious candidate for this role is the complex neural network which pervades the intestinal mucosa. The probable involvement of the autonomic nervous system in the stimulus-response pathway described by Sakata and Yajima was confirmed by the fact that the effect was abolished by surgical destruction of the vagus nerve.

There is also strong evidence that one or more hormonal factors are involved in the control of intestinal mucosal cell proliferation. For example parabiotic studies, in which the circulation of a treated animal is 'crossed' with that of an untreated individual or 'parabiont', have been used to show that surgical manipulation of the gut in the treated animal induces adaptive changes in the recipient. Similarly, within a single individual, exclusion of a length of small bowel from the normal nutrient flow leads to mucosal atrophy. However, this effect can be prevented if a substantial proportion of the remaining functionally intact intestine is removed. This phenomenon suggests that adaptation of the gut remnant leads to the release of some blood-borne factor capable of stimulating mucosal growth.

Several gastrointestinal peptides have been identified as candidate 'growth hormones'. These include gastrin and cholecystokinin, the main functions of which are the control of intestinal motility and gastric and pancreatic secretion during digestion. However, the trophic effects of these peptides seem to be of only minor importance in relation to the colon and the small bowel. A more probable candidate is enteroglucagon, a family of glucagon-like peptides known to be released from endocrine cells in the distal small intestine and proximal colon. Interest in enteroglucagon was stimulated initially by the identification of a small number of patients who exhibited mucosal hypertrophy associated with enteroglucagon-secreting tumours. The stimulus for enteroglucagon release is direct contact between enteroglucagon cells and luminal nutrients such as carbohydrates and lipids. Fermentable, non-absorbable disaccharides such as lactulose also cause the release of enteroglucagon in the rat, presumably because of stimulation of enteroglucagon cells by short-chain fatty acids produced by fermentation in the caecum and colon. High levels of enteroglucagon are consistently observed in the circulation of animals in whom the rate of mucosal cell proliferation has been stimulated by dietary treatment with various sources of dietary fibre, or by surgical resection, but this link remains circumstantial. Indeed studies with isolated mucosal cells grown *in vitro* have even suggested an antiproliferative role for enteroglucagon. The physiological role of this enigmatic blood-borne factor will probably remain an open question until significant quantities of the synthetic peptides become available.

In the present context, the importance of hormonal or neural factors in the control of mucosal cell proliferation is that these mechanisms are susceptible to a variety of different stimuli. If enteroglucagon, or some other growth-promoting hormonal factor, can be released both by nutrients in the small intestine and by the production of short chain fatty acids in the colon, then different components of dietary fibre may act through different mechanisms, and yet share a final common signal. For example, dietary lipid is known to stimulate mucosal cell proliferation (*Jenkins &*

Thompson, 1992). A delay in fat absorption caused by the presence of viscous polysaccharides in the small intestine (see Chapter 3) is likely to expose endocrine cells in the distal ileum to increased levels of intraluminal lipid. This could provide a mechanism to explain the stimulation of cell proliferation caused by non-fermentable food gums. In the case of guar gum, it may also explain the fact that the trophic effects of this viscous polysaccharide combined with a high level of dietary lipid are greater than the effect of either alone (*Pell et al., 1992*).

The mechanisms discussed so far depend on indirect effects of polysaccharides per se, or the direct effects of their breakdown products. However, certain polysaccharides appear to exert a direct effect in their own right on mucosal cell proliferation in the colon. Poligeenan is a sulphated polysaccharide, of relatively low molecular weight, derived from iota carrageenan by acid hydrolysis. It is noteworthy because prolonged feeding with this material leads to the induction of colorectal tumours in rats (*Oohashi et al., 1979*). Wilcox et al. (*1992*) have compared the pattern of colonic mucosal proliferation in rats fed poligeenan, carrageenan and guar gum. All three polysaccharides caused an increase in the activity of the enzyme thymidine kinase, which is a marker of proliferative activity. However, poligeenan was quite distinct from guar and carageenan in that it caused a significant displacement of proliferative activity toward the luminal pole of the crypts, and the abnormalities induced by poligeenan persisted after its withdrawal from the diet. Thus, poligeenan appears to act as a non-genotoxic carcinogen but its mechanism of action is not known. At present it would seem to bear no functional resemblance to any known dietary fibre.

----5.3----
MUCOSAL CELL PROLIFERATION AND COLORECTAL CARCINOGENESIS

Replication of the intestinal epithelial cells is a normal physiological process, essential to the maintenance of morphology and functional integrity throughout the gut. In animal models, stimulation of mucosal proliferation appears to aid healing and adaptation after gastrointestinal surgery. Conversely, in humans a reduction in mucosal proliferative activity, such as that associated with chronic use of some non-steroidal anti-inflammatory drugs, can lead to a reduction in the repair capabilities of the mucosa and hence an increased risk of duodenal ulcer. What then, if any, is the significance of fibre-induced changes in gastrointestinal mucosal cell proliferation for human health?

In colorectal cancer, the normal processes of cell division, differentiation, senescence and exfoliation from the colonic surface become progressively more abnormal. The earliest stages in the process are thought to be hyperproliferation of the mucosal crypt cells and a spatial displacement of mitosis away from the base of the crypt towards the mucosal surface. This effect occurs throughout the entire mucosa, but the next stage is the development of focal lesions which are thought to have their origins in single aberrant crypts. Instead of normal immature cells which cease dividing and acquire the functional characteristics of typical columnar epithelial cells, the crypt becomes filled with poorly differentiated cells which persist at the mucosal surface and continue to divide, giving rise first to an adenoma or non-invasive polyp, and eventually to a malignant tumour. In humans this process takes years but it occurs much more quickly in animals treated with chemical carcinogens. The progressive development of the tumour is associated with the acquisition of genetic abnormalities at particular alleles which are known to function as proto-oncogenes or tumour suppressor genes. The presence of these genetic lesions is thought to be fundamental to the process of tumorigenesis, although the precise role of each lesion in the induction of uncontrolled cell growth is poorly understood at present (*Fearon & Vogelstein, 1990*).

Dividing cells undergoing DNA synthesis are highly susceptible to the occurrence of mutations and gene deletions. For this reason, tissues with a high rate of cell proliferation are thought to be vulnerable to the development of cancer (*Preston-Martin et al., 1990*). Secondary bile acids are thought to stimulate cell proliferation in the colon and it has been postulated that they increase the risk of colorectal cancer by this mechanism.

A supposedly protective effect of dietary fibre against colorectal cancer is one of the best known and widely accepted aspects of the dietary fibre hypothesis. Nevertheless the epidemiological evidence for this relationship remains inconclusive and no wholly convincing protective mechanism has been established. Still less is there any firm epidemiological or experimental evidence as to the relative effectiveness of the many different types of NSP on carcinogenic mechanisms in humans. The use of experimental animals that have been treated with chemical carcinogens to explore the effects of defined polysaccharides on the induction of tumours has done little to resolve this issue. Indeed, by no means all forms of dietary fibre are protective in this model, and some may even accelerate the induction or promotion of tumours through their stimulatory effect on mucosal cell proliferation.

As with many aspects of research on dietary fibre, unambiguous conclusions are difficult to achieve because of the considerable variety of experimental conditions and types of dietary fibre which have been used by researchers. One of the most important variables appears to be the timing of treatment with dietary fibre in relation to the administration of the carcinogen. Jacobs (*1983*) administered a diet containing wheat bran (20%) to rats during the period of exposure to the carcinogen 1,2-dimethy-lhydrazine dihydrochloride (DMH) and observed a significantly higher yield of experimental tumours. In Jacobs' studies, feeding wheat bran led to increased proliferation and expansion of the proliferative compartment. This effect combined additively with the hyperproliferation caused by treatment with DMH alone, and the author proposed that the synergistic effect of dietary fibre and carcinogen stimulated tumorigenesis by enhancing initiation, promotion or both (*Jacobs, 1984*). A similar enhancement of tumour induction has been observed after chemical treatment of animals fed guar gum, pectin, oat bran or corn bran (*Jacobs, 1986*). In contrast, other workers have reported a protective effect of certain types of fibre fed to animals during the period of tumour promotion, after treatment with chemical carcinogens. For example Wilpart and Roberfroid (*1987*) administered diets containing cellulose or a commercial bulk laxative based on ispaghula husk (Fybogel®; arabinosyl rhamnosylxylan; Reckitt & Colman, UK) to rats previously treated with DMH. Under these conditions the ispaghula husk inhibited tumorigenesis whereas cellulose did not. One possible explanation is the recently recognized ability of butyrate to 'detransform' potentially cancerous mucosal cells so that, although the proliferation of normal cells so that, although the proliferation of normal cells may be enhanced, the appearance of tumour cells may be suppressed (*Scheppach et al., 1992*).

The confusion surrounding the apparently contradictory findings of different workers in this field may be partly explained by differences in the quantities as well as the type of dietary fibre used in experimental studies with animals. It has recently been reported that mucosal cell proliferation was suppressed in rats fed wheat bran at 5% of the total diet, compared to controls fed no fibre, but at 10% and 20% inclusion, hyperproliferation progressively recurred (*Boffa et al., 1992*). On the basis of this and other aspects of their results the authors proposed that, whereas a moderate amount of dietary fibre may inhibit carcinogenesis, both too much or too little may actually promote it.

——5.4——
SIGNIFICANCE FOR HUMAN HEALTH

What is the significance of these findings in relation to human health? Epidemiology is a somewhat blunt-edged tool which offers little clue as to the effects of particular NSP. In general, although the evidence for a strong protective effect of dietary fibre against colorectal cancer remains tantalizingly inconclusive, there is little evidence of any adverse effect. Even so, there has been one study which has shown a positive relationship between cereal fibre consumption and cancer of the colon in an Australian population (*Potter & McMichael, 1986*), and there is weak but long-standing evidence for a positive relationship between cereal fibre and stomach cancer (*Hakama & Saxen, 1967*). Jacobs has pointed out that several studies that have shown an inverse correlation between fibre consumption and colorectal cancer have also contained evidence for a positive relationship with gastric cancer, but the latter has rarely if ever been commented upon by the authors (*Jacobs, 1987*). It is certainly interesting to note that mortality from stomach cancer has been in long-term decline in most Western countries during the period when consumption of dietary fibre has fallen. However, no firm conclusions can be drawn from such circumstantial evidence.

Epidemiology shows that populations with a high average faecal output are at relatively low risk of colorectal cancer (*Cummings et al., 1992*). Dietary fibre is a major determinant of faecal bulk, but self-selected diets that are rich in fibre will draw upon a variety of sources, including vegetables and fruits, which seem to exert an independent protective effect against many forms of cancer. Once again we encounter the problem of distinguishing between the effects of dietary fibre per se, and the effects of the many other characteristics of fibre- rich diets. Moreover, these epidemiological findings do not prove that a diet that contains high levels of any one particular source of dietary fibre, whether consumed as a supplement, or in the form of specialized food products, will necessarily confer protective effects. It is probably only in recent times that it has become relatively easy to consume a diet that is rich both in saturated fat and in the soluble NSP that support a high rate of mucosal cell proliferation in animals. There is therefore no epidemiological evidence as yet with which to assess the long-term effects of such diets. Clearly the complex polysaccharides in our diets exert subtle effects on mucosal cell proliferation which were not suspected when the dietary fibre hypothesis was formulated. The biological basis for such effects, and their significance, if any, for health are questions which remain unresolved.

FURTHER READING

Spiller GA. *CRC Handbook of Dietary Fiber in Human Nutrition*. 2nd ed. Boca Raton: CRC Press, 1993.

Wright NA, Alison M. *The Biology of Epithelial Cell Populations*. Vols 1 & 2. Oxford: Clarendon Press, 1984.

CHAPTER
—6—

Adverse Effects of Substances Associated with Fibre

The strict definition of dietary fibre includes only NSP derived from plant cell walls. However, the sources from which these polysaccharides are derived are usually complex plant tissues containing a variety of other structural elements and secondary metabolites. The trend toward increased consumption of dietary fibre may therefore lead to a greater intake of many other substances besides complex carbohydrates. This is equally true in the case of consumers increasing their intake of unprocessed 'wholefoods' such as seed legumes, and those favouring commercial products such as breads, snack foods and breakfast cereals containing processed fibre supplements.

Many food plants contain tissues that, although intrinsically unpalatable and low in nutritional value, contain high levels of NSP. In recent years the greatly increased demand for sources of dietary fibre has encouraged the exploitation of food constituents that have not previously been regarded as useful food ingredients. Moreover, modern food processing technology has assisted this trend. For example, extrusion cooking is ideally suited to the continuous processing of complex carbohydrates with a relatively low moisture content. Granular mixtures, flours or doughs can be processed and cooked simultaneously at high temperature and pressure, and very high shear forces can be applied to alter texture and improve palatability. However, the application of such techniques could encourage the inadvertent use of novel ingredients containing antinutritional or potentially toxic factors, and this fact needs to be considered when evaluating new ingredients or developing new products.

The plant cell wall contains many non-carbohydrate components, including cutins, lignin, silica and flavonoids. There is also an almost endless list of biologically active plant constituents which, though not cell wall components per se, may be present at relatively high levels in the plant tissues that are utilized as sources of dietary fibre, and could be carried over as contaminants into food. In this chapter the properties of some of the more common substances will be briefly reviewed to illustrate the limitations they may impose on the use of plant materials as sources of dietary fibre.

------ 6.1 ------
PLANT POLYPHENOLS

The plant polyphenols, or 'vegetable tannins', are a complex group of substances distributed widely throughout the plant kingdom. They are characterized by an abundance of phenolic groups and a considerable variety of polymeric structures, with molecular weights ranging from around 3000 to 20,000 Daltons. Two principal classes exist, the proanthocyanadins, and the galloyl and the hexahydroxydiphenoyl esters. The salient functional property of these compounds is the ability to form irreversible complexes with proteins. Tannins derived from oak bark or galls have been used since prehistoric times to cross-link the collagen fibrils of animal hides, thereby turning them into leather, which is characteristically tough and resistant to microbial degradation. Polyphenols are secondary plant metabolites with no apparent function in plant physiology. They do however reduce the palatability of plant tissues to herbivores, and they are probably toxic to microbes and invertebrates. For human beings the formation of complexes with glycoproteins of the oropharyngeal mucosae leads to the characteristic sensation of dryness and superficial 'tightness' known as astringency. When controlled and nurtured, this effect of tannins is one of the prized virtues of a properly made red wine.

The significance of plant polyphenols from the point of view of human nutrition is rather limited, but they are important as a source of flavour and 'character' in many foods and beverages besides wine. Infusions such as tea and coffee contain substantial quantities of tannins and related compounds, and these are among the most effective inhibitors of iron absorption in the human diet. The ability to interact with proteins also enables polyphenols to inhibit the activity of bacterial and mammalian enzymes. The phenolic constituents of plant cell walls have been shown to inhibit the activity of ruminal bacteria *in vitro* (*Varel & Jung, 1986*) and they may limit the utilization of forage feeds by cattle and other ruminants (*Jung & Fahey, 1983*). Similarly the degradation of dietary fibre in the human colon may be reduced by the presence of cell wall polyphenolics. This is particularly true in the case of wheat bran, so in this sense these compounds can be said to influence faecal bulking. Isolated phenolic compounds have also been shown to inhibit the digestibility of protein and lipids in the rat (*Nyman & Björck, 1989*).

Polyphenolic compounds in foods and beverages may also interact strongly with the superficial proteins of the alimentary tract, and thereby give rise to chronic irritation. Morton (*1970*) has made a strong case for tannins as a factor in the aetiology of oesophageal cancer. However, this disease has a very complex geographical distribution throughout the world, and it is certainly multifactorial in origin. It is unlikely that plant polyphenols are a significant cause of oesophageal cancer in the industrialized West. However, so-called 'bird-proof' sorghum, which has an exceptionally high content of polyphenols, may be a contributory factor in some regions of Africa.

A list of human food plants containing substantial quantities of polyphenols is given in Table 6.1. It is evident that polyphenols are likely to form a substantial proportion of the non-digestible fraction of fruit pulps, and the residues of such materials as cocoa bean and carob. The composition of 'dietary fibre' prepared from such materials and the biological properties of its phenolic constituents need to be carefully evaluated before they are exploited for human consumption.

Table 6.1 Some common plant foods containing significant quantities of polyphenols

Plant	Proanthocyanadins	Galloyl and hexahydroxydiphenoyl esters
Barley	•	
Sorghum	•	
Cocoa	•	
Carob		•
Guava		•
Rhubarb	•	•
Persimmon	•	•
Apple	•	
Pear	•	
Currant	•	
Strawberry	•	•
Raspberry	•	•
Grape	•	

——6.2——
SAPONINS AND GLYCOALKALOIDS

Saponins are another group of secondary plant metabolites that are thought to play a role as natural pesticides, and are distributed so widely throughout the plant kingdom that they inevitably occur in a variety of human foods. They have long been recognized for their 'soaplike' surfactant properties, and for their toxicity, especially to invertebrates and fishes. The characteristic structure of saponins comprises a lipophilic aglycone, which can be either a steroid or a triterpenoid, and one or more hydrophilic sugar chains. This structure accounts for the amphipathic properties of the group, and for their ability to form complexes with sterols, including those of cellular membranes. Thus saponins give rise to foam in aqueous solution, and cause lysis of erythrocytes and other mammalian cells, two properties which have long been used as qualitative chemical tests for their presence in plant tissues.

Saponins are a normal constituent of the human diet. They are not particularly closely associated with plant cell walls, but they are plentiful in certain foods which are often advocated as good sources of dietary fibre. In a recent study it has been shown that baked beans are the main source of saponins among omnivorous consumers in the UK, and that the most common type consumed are soy saponins (*Ridout et al., 1988*). Soy saponins have been shown to be mildly membranolytic towards intestinal mucosal cells *in vitro* (*Johnson et al., 1986*), but there is no evidence that they are in any way injurious to health. This is not necessarily true of other saponins found in plants used as human foods. The introduction of exotic ingredients from relatively remote cultures and cuisines is an increasingly common feature of Western food production and marketing. Quinoa is a case in point. This robust high-protein crop has been used for millennia as a staple food in the highlands of South America, and the seeds are now being marketed in North America and Western Europe as a novel source of vegetable protein. Of the different varieties of quinoa that are used as food, some are high in bitter, membranolytic saponins, which are toxic. The traditional technique for removing the saponins is prolonged washing in flowing water. 'Sweet' varieties of quinoa do exist but for most purposes the saponins must be removed by washing and processing on a commercial scale before the product can be made wholesome and safe for human consumption. The possibility that exotic plant foods contain saponins is one of the issues that must be considered before they are introduced as a major component of human diets, and this is particularly true of legume seeds which may be selected for their high fibre content. Some common foods known to contain saponins are listed in Table 6.2.

The common glycoalkaloids found in the human diet are alpha-solanine and alpha-chaconine, both of which are found in potatoes, and alpha-tomatine, which is a constituent of green tomatoes. They share many of the structural and chemical properties of saponins, including the capacity to form complexes with membrane sterols. In the present context, the most remarkable property of the glycoalkaloids is their

Table 6.2 Some common human plant foods known to contain significant quantities of saponins

Soya beans
Kidney and other beans (*Phaseolus sp.*)
Guar beans and pods (*Cyamopsis*)
Tomato
Onion
Asparagus
Spinach
Sugar beet
Alfalfa
Blackberry
Fenugreek
Liquorice

toxicity, which is comparable to that of strychnine, and quite exceptional for such a common dietary constituent.

Low concentrations of glycoalkaloids are present throughout the potato plant, but they reach high levels in potato tubers during sprouting, and as a defensive response to damage or infestation. They are therefore most abundant in old or damaged potatoes. Even good quality tubers contain a significant quantity, particularly in the skin and underlying tissue. Peeling and boiling reduces the glycoalkaloid content of the tubers but some is inevitably consumed. It has been calculated that the average daily intake of glycoalkaloids is only a factor of about five times lower than the toxic dose for man. This is a remarkably small margin of safety, and it is perhaps surprising that only a few authenticated cases of glycoalkaloid poisoning have been reported.

It is often assumed that most of the dietary fibre content of potatoes is associated with the skins, and that consumption of potatoes cooked in their 'jackets' is beneficial. In fact, the presence or absence of the skin makes relatively little difference to the fibre content of the potato, and the physiological effects of suberin, the major constituent of the skin, are unknown. However, consumption of potato skins does seem likely to increase the dietary intake of glycoalkaloids and it seems doubtful whether the practice should be encouraged. If skins must be used for culinary purposes they should be of the highest quality, and they must not be stored or processed in such a way as to favour the accumulation of glycoalkaloids.

———6.3———
LECTINS

Many of the most potent of all natural toxins found in plants belong to a very large group of proteins, the lectins. As with the substances discussed previously, the lectins are widely distributed throughout the plant kingdom, but they are remarkable for their highly specific biological activity against animal cells. Unlike the saponins, which cause a non-specific lysis of erythrocytes, lectins cause them to aggregate into clumps. This process of agglutination gives rise to the synonyms 'phytoagglutins' and 'phytohaemagglutinins'. The biological effects of lectins are caused by their ability to bind specifically to the sugar groups of cell membrane glycoproteins, which, in the case of erythrocytes, are often the same receptors that define blood group specificity. Lectins are in no sense a component of dietary fibre but they are often present in high concentrations in foods that might be expected to form an important part of a high-fibre diet. Concanavalin A (con A) is a well-known lectin derived from the jack bean (*Canavalia ensiformis*). This seed is not used as a human food. However, a graphic description of the effects of ingesting just 10 mg of purified con A in water has been given by Freed (1987). Gastrointestinal symptoms including colic, flatus, abnormal bowel habit and passage of mucus were experienced for a period of 3 days.

Clearly the cells lining the gastrointestinal tract are the first target for dietary lectins. The effects on the gut of lectins derived from raw kidney beans (*Phaseolus vulgaris*) have been studied extensively using experimental animals (*Pusztai et al., 1986*). Within 10 days of feeding raw kidney bean protein or pure lectins the small intestinal mucosal mass is doubled, despite the fact that the villi become stunted. The extra mass is due to hyperproliferation of the crypt cells, presumably in response to destruction of enterocytes by lectins which become bound to the brush border and incorporated into the cell interior. There is also a general decline in mucosal function, an increase in mucosal permeability, a loss of serum proteins to the intestinal lumen and increased mucus production, all of which contribute to loss of nitrogen in the faeces and impaired nutrition (*Greer & Pusztai, 1985*).

The effects of lectins are not confined to the mucosal cells of the alimentary tract. Pusztai and his colleagues (*1986*) have reported that in rats as much as 10% of an ingested dose of kidney bean lectin is absorbed into the circulation in a form giving rise to a specific immunoglobulin G type antibody response. Moreover, the specific interaction of some lectins with cells of the immune system enables them to modulate the proliferation and activity of T and B lymphocytes, and hence to stimulate or suppress immune activity, depending on the experimental conditions. Other possible systemic targets for ingested lectins include the epithelial cells of the kidney tubules, nerve cells and insulin receptors. The range of pathological effects that dietary lectins might, in principle, bring about is therefore immense. It should not however be assumed that the biological effects of lectins are necessarily all injurious to health. Some have been shown to exhibit antitumour activity *in vitro* , and it has been proposed that dietary lectins may protect against cancer of the colon

(*Freed & Green, 1975*). However, this hypothesis remains untested.

What is the overall significance of dietary lectins for human health and what, if any, is the connection with dietary fibre? It needs to be emphasized that lectins are very common in the human diet (Table 6.3). So widely distributed are they that human beings must have become adapted to their presence in foods over a very substantial period of evolutionary history. Many lectins are undoubtedly harmless, and some may be beneficial to health. One example is the tomato lectin, which is commonly ingested from raw tomatoes, and is known to be both biologically active and resistant to digestion. There is very strong epidemiological evidence suggesting that tomatoes and other raw salad fruits and vegetables contribute to the maintenance of health. On the other hand changes in

Table 6.3 Some common human foods with significant lectin activity *in vitro*

Vegetables
    Tomato[a]
    Potato[a]
    Carrot[a]
    Turnip[b]
    Radish[b]
    Sweet peppers[b]
    Celery[b]
    Green peas[a]
    Kidney beans[a]
    (Many other varieties of *Phaseolus vulgaris*)[b]
Fruits
    Apples[b]
    Grapefruit[b]
    Lemon[b]
    Orange[b]
    Banana[b]
    Strawberry[b]
    Raspberries[a]
    Grapes[a]
Cereals and cereal products
    Maize[b]
    Rice[b]
    Barley[b]
    Wheat germ[a]
    Corn Flakes[a]
    All Bran[a]
    Shredded Wheat[a]

[a] Data obtained by Nachbar & Oppenheim (*1980*)
[b] Data quoted from other sources in Nachbar & Oppenheim (*1980*)

dietary fashion and culinary practice can spring some surprises. The popularity of relatively unprocessed 'wholefoods' and vegetarian diets, coupled with the growing abundance of imported foods in prosperous societies, may expose populations to very high intakes of novel lectins. Judging by the list of foods in Table 6.3, the dietary fibre hypothesis has probably contributed to this trend.

Perhaps the most famous toxic hazard caused by dietary lectins is poisoning by undercooked kidney beans, which leads to severe gastrointestinal symptoms (*Noah et al., 1980*). Kidney bean lectins retain their activity after 4 hours of cooking at 70° C, and even boiling for 45 minutes is not entirely effective as a means of destroying their activity unless they have previously been soaked for several hours. Legumes are rich in dietary fibre, and particularly the soluble components which have been advocated for the management of diabetes mellitus. Clearly the possible hazards of such diets need to be understood and avoided by careful culinary practice.

——6.4——
PHYTIC ACID

Phytic acid, myo-inositol hexaphosphate, is commonly found in foods in association with the plant cell wall and is therefore one of the 'associated substances' most frequently mentioned in discussions on the physiological effects of dietary fibre (*Frølich, 1992*). In the plant the phytic acid is usually present as the mixed salts with potassium, magnesium and calcium and one should therefore more correctly refer to the 'phytates' in foods. Inositol hexaphosphate contains about 28.1% phosphorus, and it functions in the plant as a storage compound for inorganic phosphate ions which are used in the energy metabolism of the plant, especially during germination.

As one would expect from their physiological role in the plant, phytates are found in the greatest concentrations in seed tissues. The highest concentrations therefore occur in foods such as cereal grains and their products, in nuts and in seed legumes. Generally speaking the concentrations are lower in other plant foods. Within the tissues of the seed, the phytates are localized at sites that will be most metabolically active at germination. Table 6.4 illustrates this by showing values for phytic acid in some typical foods. The values in the table are taken from Holland, Unwin and Buss (*1988; 1991; 1992*) and are based on data originally published in McCance and Widdowson (*1960*).

Cereals

The highest amounts of phytates are found in wheat germ, wheat bran and other high-extraction cereal foods, such as wholewheat breakfast cereals and wholemeal bread. In most other cooked and prepared cereal foods the concentrations are usually less than 100 mg/100 g.

Vegetables

Most vegetables contain levels of the order of 10–80 mg/100 g, but the seed legumes are an important exception. Although the dried beans contain levels of the order of 700–1300 mg/100 g, the concentrations fall to the order of 200–300 mg/100 g when they are cooked and ready for consumption. Potatoes tend to have higher levels than green vegetables, with new potatoes having about 80 mg/100 g.

Fruits

The phytate concentrations of fruits are low around 10-30 mg/100 g.

Nuts

As one should expect on physiological grounds, the phytate values in nuts are similar to whole cereal grains, ranging from about 600 mg in walnuts to 3000 mg in sunflower seeds.

6.4.1 Physiological Effects in Humans

Phytic acid combines with inorganic cations to form salts. The salts of calcium, iron and zinc are insoluble, and the classical studies of McCance and Widdowson in the 1940s showed that the adverse effects of high-extraction wheat products such as wholemeal bread on human mineral metabolism could be attributed to the high levels of phytate that were complexing with the calcium and iron in the diet. As these complexes were insoluble they were excreted in the faeces (*McCance & Widdowson, 1942*). Studies with rats did not show such strong effects, however. This is probably due to the presence of phytases in the small intestine, enzymes which hydrolyse the phytates, releasing the bound cations. The phytases do not appear to be endogenous in origin but are more likely to be due to bacterial contamination of the upper gastrointestinal tract, which is common in rats because of coprophagy. This is also seen in the pig, in which the bacterial counts in the small intestine are much higher than those in man.

In experimental studies where phytates have been fed in conjunction with dietary fibre from cereals it has been shown that the lower absorption of calcium and iron from these diets is virtually entirely attributable to the phytate, although some residual non-phytate effects are evident with zinc (*British Nutrition Foundation, 1990*). In a major review of the evidence for effects in humans, Rossander and colleagues (*1992*) reached a similar conclusion, drawing on results from studies with ileostomists (see Chapter 4), and from studies where the plant foods had been treated with phytases to hydrolyse the phytates. Nevertheless many rural African populations appear to absorb calcium quite well from high-phytate diets. This raises the possibility that some adaptive mechanism may exist which overcomes the adverse effects on mineral metabolism in populations chronically exposed to them. However, studies with human subjects have failed to show that it is possible to induce phytase activity by feeding high levels of phytate.

Some authors have suggested that the capacity of phytate to bind iron in the gastrointestinal tract may have positive benefits in that it prevents the unabsorbed inorganic iron acting as a generator of free radicals. These short-lived but highly reactive chemical species are capable of inflicting considerable damage on living cells, including the induction of mutations by direct damage to DNA. An accumulation of genetic defects is associated with the development of colorectal cancer, and it has been proposed that the presence of free iron in the gut lumen may accelerate this process. At the present time this hypothesis remains somewhat speculative, although it does illustrate a principle that many natural components of foods may have both beneficial and adverse effects. It is essential to understand the balance of these opposing phenomena, and one must avoid thinking about the constituents of food in too simplistic a fashion.

6.4.2 Effects of Food Processing on Phytates

Many of the workers in the field of mineral nutrition feel that it would be advantageous to reduce the phytate levels in high-extraction cereal foods, which are potentially rich sources of several inorganic nutrients. This could be done by encouraging the use of traditional fermentation processes which have always been widely used in food preparation. Thus the traditional bread-making process results in considerable reductions in the phytate concentration in the bread compared with the starting flour. This is also true for fermented soya products such as tofu. These processes use the endogenous enzymes in the plant foods themselves or in the yeasts. The addition of exogenous phytases, while being technologically attractive, would involve considerable effort in safety evaluation. Extrusion cooking does not reduce phytate levels, probably because the high temperatures inactivate the endogenous phytases before they can act.

Hydrolysis of the phytates produces a range of phosphates, ranging down to the inositol monophosphates. It is interesting to note that some of these promote the absorption of iron, possibly by chelation effects similar to those seen with ascorbate and citrate (*Sandberg et al., 1989*).

FURTHER READING

British Nutrition Foundation. *Complex Carbohydrates in Foods.* London: Chapman & Hall, 1990, pp 39–44.

Freed DLJ. Dietary lectins and disease. In: *Food Allergy and Intolerance.* Brostoff J, Challacombe SJ, eds. London: Baillière Tindall, 1987.

Frølich, W. Bioavailability of minerals from cereals. In: *Handbook of Dietary Fiber in Human Nutrition,* 2nd ed. Spiller GA, ed. Boca Raton: CRC Press, 1992, pp 209–52.

Haslam E. *Plant Polyphenols.* Cambridge: Cambridge University Press, 1980.

Holland B, Unwin ID, Buss DH. *Cereals and Cereal Products.* Cambridge: Royal Society of Chemistry and MAFF, 1988.

Holland B, Unwin ID, Buss DH. *Vegetables, Herbs and Spices.* Cambridge: Royal Society of Chemistry and MAFF, 1991.

Holland B, Unwin ID, Buss DH. *Fruits and Nuts.* Cambridge: Royal Society of Chemistry and MAFF, 1992.

Price KR, Johnson IT, Fenwick GR. The chemistry and biological significance of saponins in foods and feedingstuffs. *Crit Rev Food Sci Nutr* 1987; 26: 27–135.

CHAPTER

—7—

Toxicological and Regulatory Aspects of Dietary Fibre

The growth of public interest in the dietary fibre hypothesis as promoted in the lectures and writings of Burkitt and Trowell in the early 1970s led to a public demand for high-fibre foods, and this encouraged food producers and retailers to produce and promote both existing and modified products claiming to be good sources of dietary fibre. Two general strategies can be adopted by consumers wishing to increase their intake of fibre. The first approach is to increase the consumption of foods containing abundant quantities of cell wall polysaccharides as original structural components. Such foods include many vegetables and fruits, and of course high-extraction cereal products of a traditional type. These foods are already familiar to most of us and it is simply their variety and relative proportions in the diet which need to be modified. This approach has often been favoured by advisory bodies such as NACNE in setting dietary recommendations for the UK population. The second strategy is to consume foods in which the dietary fibre content has been increased by the food manufacturer, using modern processing techniques to incorporate supplements based on NSP or, perhaps, resistant starch. Such foods have proved popular with many consumers who wish to increase their intake of dietary fibre for health reasons, but to whom diets with a high content of vegetables and high-extraction cereals may be unattractive or inconvenient. They are also popular with food manufacturers who seek to meet consumer demands and introduce new 'added value' products into the marketplace. Most consumers probably adopt a middle course, but demand for new products containing a high proportion of dietary fibre is likely to continue, and food manufacturers will search for novel ingredients having the appropriate functionality and palatability. In this chapter we will consider the definition and analysis of fibre for regulatory and labelling purposes and the practicality and need for toxicological evaluation of such ingredients.

——7.1——
NUTRITIONAL LABELLING

In late 1978 a review of the nutritional aspects of bread and flour was started in the UK (*Department of Health and Social Security, 1981*), which recommended, among other matters, that breads should be labelled with their dietary fibre content to enable the consumer to choose a high-fibre product. This led in turn to a review of the possible analytical approaches for the measurement of dietary fibre for the purposes of labelling of breads. In the USA a parallel development arose from the recommendations of the McGovern report (*US Senate Select Committee on Nutrition & Human Needs, 1977*), which had recommended an increased intake of complex carbohydrate foods. As public interest in dietary fibre grew in the USA, moves toward the identification of a regulatory method for the analysis of dietary fibre were led by the Association of Official Analytical Chemists (AOAC). Both these activities had a similar aim but the approaches differed, largely because of the way that carbohydrate analysis had developed in the two countries.

In the UK there was a long analytical tradition of measuring carbohydrates which had been begun by McCance and Lawrence (*1929*). There was therefore a natural focus on the chemical analysis of the constituent polysaccharides as a method for establishing the dietary fibre levels in foods. The evolution of the non-starch polysaccharide (NSP) method, which was eventually adopted by the Ministry of Agriculture, Fisheries and Food (MAFF) for nutritional labelling in the UK (*MAFF, 1992*) has been described in Chapter 2. At the present time the provision of fibre values, and indeed of all nutritional labelling, is voluntary, although, when used, the format should follow the guidance from MAFF (*1987*).

In the USA, carbohydrates had customarily been measured by difference: that is, by measuring water, protein (calculated from total nitrogen multiplied by a factor), fat and ash, and deducting the sum of these from 100 to give a carbohydrate value. Crude fibre was also measured gravimetrically by the traditional Weende method, much modified technically to improve its performance. Those advising the AOAC felt that a gravimetric method would be preferable because it used simple apparatus and was not particularly demanding on technical skills. (Incidentally, this view does not reflect the very real technical difficulties entailed in performing the classical crude fibre method.) The analytical focus therefore was to measure dietary fibre as the indigestible material in foods, albeit with a final correction for indigestible protein and ash. This approach led to the development of the AOAC total dietary fibre (TDF) method which has also been described in Chapter 2 (*Prosky et al., 1984*). This gravimetric method measures the NSP together with lignin and lignin-like artefacts, and resistant starch, plus all other insoluble components not removed during the enzymatic stages. It thus gives higher values than the NSP method advocated by the UK MAFF.

The controversy over the choice of method for nutritional labelling of foods for their fibre content has been brought into sharper focus because of the proposal to implement Nutritional Labelling in the European Community (1992). In these discussions several member countries favour the AOAC gravimetric approach. Also, because the method gives higher values, it tends to be favoured by the producers of high-fibre products who naturally prefer to have the higher value for use on their product labels. This, together with the apparently lower capital and staff resources required for the AOAC method, are proving very influential at the time of writing (1993). It should be noted, however, that both methods have relatively low precision, and neither provides a direct prediction of biological effect or benefit. The quality control of dietary fibre analyses requires the development and use of Certified Standard Reference Materials and these are under development at the present time. Nevertheless the challenge of devising an analytical technique which accurately reflects the behaviour of cell wall polysaccharides in the gut lumen during digestion remains to be met.

7.1.1 Problems Posed by Novel Polysaccharides

In the original hypothesis the term 'dietary fibre' was used for the plant cell wall materials in foods. Isolated polysaccharides were included in the definition for pragmatic reasons and because they were virtually all derived initially from plant cell walls (see Chapter 1). The use of indigestibility as the criterion for distinguishing dietary fibre from other polysaccharides has led to several indigestible polysaccharides and higher oligosaccharides being loosely described and promoted as dietary fibre ingredients. These have included the semisynthetic glucan Polydextrose® (Pfizer Chemicals) and analogous compounds, and the fructan inulin. There are in addition a large number of potential semisynthetic polysaccharides under development at the present time which are indigestible in the sense that they do not contain alpha-glucosidic links and will therefore not be hydrolysed in the small intestine. Moreover, it is possible to imagine the development of resistant starches that could be included in this category.

Neither the AOAC TDF procedure nor the NSP methods measure these types of compound completely, so in formal technical terms they cannot be regarded as dietary fibre. Moreover, from the viewpoint of the original hypothesis, and on the basis of epidemiological evidence about the protective effects of diets containing plant cell wall material, there is good reason to exclude these compounds from fibre declarations on conceptual grounds as well. If, as some would advocate, the definition of dietary fibre is simplified to that of indigestibility alone, then there are logical arguments for including all indigestible components of the diet. However, this approach is at variance with the original concept of dietary fibre, and in effect would entail a new hypothesis that the amount of indigestible matter in a diet, regardless of its origin or composition, is responsible for protective effects. There is at present no evidence for such a hypothesis.

—7.2—
TOXICOLOGICAL AND NUTRITIONAL EVALUATION OF FIBRE PREPARATIONS

Although there are complex health issues associated with any major change in dietary composition, the issue of safety evaluation does not usually arise in relation to traditional foods with a high fibre content. However, purified NSP intended for use as food supplements may be classified as food additives by regulatory bodies, and a complete formal toxicological evaluation may be required. The evaluation of a dietary fibre preparation must, like that of any of any novel food or component of foods, be considered under two headings (*Department of Health, 1991*). The first is the conventional one of safety. Under this heading one would need to consider the overall specification of the preparation, including the bacterial and fungal contamination of the product, and especially the possible presence of mycotoxins. The plant source from which the preparation was obtained would also have to be considered as there would, as we have seen earlier, be the possibility of natural toxicants being present, possibly at higher levels than in the starting material due to the extraction process used in preparing the high-fibre material.

Toxicological evaluation of an ingredient, rather than an additive or a component added at low levels, is more difficult because techniques devised for the evaluation of substances incorporated into foods at low concentrations may not lend themselves to bulk constituents. For example, one cannot simply feed such constituents at grossly increased levels without distorting the dietary intake of the test animals. In many cases therefore any evidence for adverse effects has to rely on careful chemical analysis, and evidence deduced from a thorough nutritional evaluation.

The nutritional evaluation is the second element of the assessment. This involves feeding trials where the effects on food intake, body weight, and other nutritional parameters are carefully measured. In particular, the effects on mineral availability would need to be investigated using conventional balance studies, and more acute studies of absorption from meals would be carried out using radio- or stable isotopes. The animals would normally be fed at levels likely to be used in the human diet, and at also at increased levels, although, as previously mentioned, problems with distortion of the dietary intake are likely to occur.

Once conventional safety is established, controlled human studies would, in some cases, be essential, for example, where effects on body weight or on serum cholesterol levels were expected, and where animal models are inadequate. These studies require careful clinical supervision and any allergic responses to the preparation would be noted. Finally a full nutritional evaluation must consider what impact the general use of the preparation might have on the nutritional value of the national diet, and on the diets of any particular target populations such as slimmers or diabetic patients who might be particularly vulnerable. The final approval requires the satisfactory integration of all these different types of evidence. Clearly safety concerns would eliminate a preparation at an early stage, as would the occurrence of allergic responses in a significant number of individuals. Adverse effects on mineral absorption would preclude the use of the ingredient in infant or toddler foods, and possibly completely.

A number of hydrocolloid gums have already been subjected to toxicological evaluation because of their original intended use as modifiers of food texture. Guar gum provides an interesting example of such a material. The cluster bean (*Cyamopsis tetragonoloba* and *C. proraloides*) is a traditional food in the Indian subcontinent, and is obtainable from Asian markets in the UK and elsewhere. The usefulness of the galactomannan gum, which functions as a storage polysaccharide in mature seeds of *Cyamopsis sp.*, was recognized by Western food manufacturers during the postwar period, and the gum now has a major role as a thickener and stabilizer of food systems. The Joint FAO/WHO Expert Committee of Food Additives agreed upon a temporary acceptable daily intake of 125 mg/kg body weight for guar gum in 1970, and the material was among a number of hydrocolloid gums classified in 1972 as 'generally recognized as safe' (GRAS) by the Subcommittee on Review of the GRAS List, under the auspices of the National Research Council and National Academy of Sciences of the USA. These findings were based on various published feeding studies with experimental animals carried out during the 1960s, and on specially commissioned mutagenicity and teratogenicity tests which demonstrated no adverse effects of guar.

Graham et al. (*1981*) subsequently undertook extended feeding trials with guar gum to determine its subacute toxicity in the rat. Even at levels as high as 15% by weight only minor signs of pathology were observed. In an acute trial it was estimated that the LD_{50} dose lay between 6 and 9 g/kg body weight. Although such studies have provided reassurance that guar gum possesses no unexpected toxic activity, hindsight demonstrates that they were unable to predict both the benefits, and the potential problems, associated with the use of guar gum as a form of dietary fibre. The ability of guar to reduce plasma cholesterol levels and attenuate postprandial blood glucose peaks in humans was not revealed by the early chronic or acute feeding trials with experimental animals, and nor were the striking effects on cell proliferation in the intestinal mucosa.

More seriously, the risk of oesophageal obstruction was not recognized until after the development and marketing of products containing the material. At the present time the GRAS approval for guar extends only to defined uses as a thickener or emulsifier. According to FDA recommendations, products marketed as slimming aids must not contain more than 0.5% guar gum, and bulk laxatives containing more than this amount must carry a warning label.

Earlier in the book it was stated that, while it has been difficult to establish with certainty that a low consumption of dietary fibre plays a causative role in the aetiology of any disease, a great deal of new knowledge about the physiology of the alimentary tract has been generated by the dietary fibre hypothesis over the last two decades. It should now be obvious to the reader that the seemingly inert plant polysaccharides which resist digestion in the proximal gut can exert a host of important physiological effects. The rational safety evaluation of new forms of non-starch polysaccharide intended for human consumption must surely draw upon this new body of knowledge, rather than adhere to standardized protocols originally intended for food additives and other industrial chemicals. For example, it is of little practical value to learn that the oral LD_{50} dose for guar gum in the rat is equivalent to an intake of around 500 g for a human being, but it may prove to be of some importance that this polysaccharide stimulates mucosal cell proliferation throughout the alimentary tract of the rat when fed at a level equivalent to only 25 g a day in humans.

The future evaluation of novel types of dietary fibre will need to begin with a rational consideration of their origin, chemical composition and physical properties, in the light of all that has been learned about the gastrointestinal tract in the years since the inception of the fibre hypothesis. The possible presence of natural toxins and other biologically active substances derived from plant residues must be considered, as must the possibility that the polysaccharide has undergone chemical degradation or modification during processing.

FURTHER READING

Department of Health. Guidelines on the Assessment of Novel Foods and Processes. Report on Health and Social Subjects, No. 38. London: HMSO, 1991.

Department of Health and Social Security. Nutritional Aspects of Bread and Flour. Report on Health and Social Subjects, No. 23. London: HMSO, 1981.

Ministry of Agriculture, Fisheries and Food. Guidelines on Nutritional Labelling. London: MAFF, 1987.

Roberfroid, M. Toxicological evaluation of dietary fibre. *Fd Chem Toxic* 1990; 28: 747–9.

References

Ahlman H. Oesophageal obstruction after intake of a health food prepration. *Lakartidningen* 1982; 79: 1479.

Albersheim P. Biogenesis of the plant cell wall. In: *Plant Biochemistry*. Bonner J, Varner JE, eds. New York: Academic Press, 1965, pp 298–321.

Allen-Mersh T, De Jode LR. Is bran useful in diverticular disease? *Br Med J* 1982; 284: 740. (Letter)

Asp NG, Johansson CG. Dietary fibre analysis. Reviews in Clinical Nutrition. *Nut Abs Rev* 1984; 54: 735–52

Asp N-G, Johansson C-G, Hallmer H, Siljestrom M. Rapid enzymatic analysis of insoluble and soluble dietary fiber. *J Food Agric Chem* 1983; 31: 476–82.

Asp N-G, Schweizer TF, Southgate DAT, Theander O. Dietary fibre analysis. In: *Dietary Fibre: A Component of Food*. Schweizer TF, Edwards, CA, eds. London: Springer Verlag, 1992, pp 57–101.

Berger M, Venhaus A. Dietary fibre in the prevention and treatment of diabetes mellitus. In: *Dietary Fibre: A Component of Food*. Schweizer TF, Edwards CA, eds. London: Springer Verlag, 1992, pp 279–93

Blackburn NA, Redfern JS, Jarjis H, Holgate AM, Hanning I, Scarpello JHB, Johnson IT, Read NW. The mechanism of action of guar gum in improving glucose tolerance in man. *Clin Sci* 1984; 52: 371–80.

Boffa LC, Lupton JR, Mariani MR, Ceppi M, Newmark HL, Scalmatti A, Lipkin M. Modulation of colonic epithelial cell proliferation, histone acetylation and luminal short chain fatty acids by variation of dietary fiber (wheat bran) in rats. *Cancer Res* 1992; 52: 5906–12.

British Nutrition Foundation. *Complex Carbohydrates in Foods*. London: Chapman & Hall, 1990, pp 39–44.

Brown NJ, Worldling J, Rumsey RDE, Read NW. The effect of guar gum on the distribution of a radiolabelled meal in the gastrointestinal tract of the rat. *Br J Nutr* 1988; 59: 223–31.

Bueno L, Praddaude F, Fioramonti J, Ruckebush Y. Effect of dietary fibre on gastrointestinal motility and jejunal transit time. *Gastroenterol* 1981; 80: 701–7.

Burkitt DP, Trowell HC, eds. *Refined Carbohydrate Foods: Some Implications of Dietary Fibre.* London: Academic Press, 1975.

Cassidy MM, Lightfoot FG, Grau LE, Story JA, Kritchevsky D, Vahouny, GV. Effect of chronic intake of dietary fibers on the ultrastructural topography of rat jejunum and colon: a scanning electron microscope study. *Am J Clin Nutr* 1981; 34: 218–28.

Cooper SG, Tracey EJ. Small bowel obstruction caused by oat bran bezoar. *New Engl J Med* 1989; 320: 1148–9.

Cummings JH, Bingham SA, Heaton KW, Eastwood MA. Fecal weight, colon cancer risk, and dietary intake of nonstarch polysaccharides (dietary fibre). *Gastroenterol* 1992; 103: 1783–9.

Department of Health. *Dietary Reference Values for Food Energy and Nutrients for the United Kingdom.* London: HMSO, 1991.

Department of Health and Social Security. *Nutritional Aspects of Bread and Flour.* Reports on Health and Social Subjects, No. 23. London, HMSO, 1981.

Dirks P, Freeman HJ. Effects of differing purified cellulose, pectin and hemicellulose fibre diets on mucosal morphology in the rat small and large intestine. *Clin Invest Med* 1987; 10: 32–8.

Eastwood MA. Dietary fibre and serum lipids. *Lancet* 1969; ii: 1222–5.

Eastwood MA, Morris EJ. Physical properties of dietary fibre that influence physiological function: A model for polymers along the gastrointestinal tract. *Am J Clin Nutr* 1991

Edstrom S, Petterson G. Oesophageal rupture after intake of a natural medicine. *Lakartidningen* 1982; 79: 1478.

Englyst HN, Cummings JH. Improved method for measurement of dietary fiber as non-starch polysaccharides in plant foods. *J Assoc Offic Analytl Chem* 1988; 71: 808–14.

Englyst HN, Wiggins HS, Cummings JH. Determination of the non-starch polysaccharides in plant foods by gas-liquid chromatography of constituent sugars as the alditol acetates. *Analyst* 1982; 107: 307–18.

Fearon ER, Vogelstein B. A genetic model for colorectal tumorigenesis. *Cell* 1990; 6: 759–67.

Freed DLJ. Dietary lectins and disease. In: *Food Allergy and Intolerance.* Brostoff J, Challacombe SJ, eds. London: Baillière Tindall, 1987.

Freed DLJ, Green FHY. Do dietary lectins protect against bowel cancer? *Lancet* 1975; ii: 371.

FrøhlichW. Bioavailability of minerals from cereals. In: *Handbook of Dietary Fiber in Human Nutrition.* 2nd ed. Spiller GA, ed. Boca Raton: CRC Press, 1992, pp 209–42.

FrøhlichW, Schweizer TF, Asp N-G. Minerals and phytate in the analysis of dietary fiber from cereals II *Cereal Chem* 1984; 61: 357–9.

Gillooly M, Bothwell TH, Torrance JD, Macphail,AP, Derman DP, Bezwoda WR, Mills W, Charlton RW, Mayet F. Effects of organic acids, phytates and polyphenols on the absorption of iron from vegetables. *Br J Nutr* 1983; 49: 331–42.

Goering HK, Van Soest PJ. Forage fiber analyses (Apparatus, reagents, procedures and some applications). US Dept Agric Handbook No. 379. Washington: US Dept Agric, 1970.

Goodlad RA, Ratcliffe B, Fordham JP, Wright NA. Does dietary fibre stimulate intestinal epithelial cell proliferation in germ free rats? *Gut* 1989; 30: 820–5.

Goodlad RA, Wright NA. Effects of addition of kaolin or cellulose to an elemental diet on intestinal cell proliferation in the mouse. *Br J Nutr* 1983; 50: 91–8

Gordon DT. *Proceedings of the Vahouny Fiber Conference, 1992.* (1994, in press.)

Graham SL, Arnold A, Kasza L, Ruffin GE, Jackson RC, Watkins TL, Graham CH. Subchronic effects of guar gum in rats. *Fd Cosmet Toxicol.* 1981; 19: 287–90

Greer F, Pusztai A. Toxicity of kidney bean (Phaseolus vulgaris) in rats: Changes in intestinal permeability. *Digestion* 1985; 32: 42–6.

Gregory J, Foster K, Tyler H, Wiseman M. *The Dietary and Nutritional Survey of British Adults.* London: HMSO, 1990.

Haber GB, Heaton KW, Murphy D, Burroughs LF. Depletion and disruption of dietary fibre, effect on satiety, plasma glucose and serum insulin. *Lancet* 1977; ii: 679–82.

Hakama M, Saxen EA. Cereal consumption and gastric cancer. *Int J Cancer* 1967; 2: 265–8.

Halama WH, Mauldin JL. Distal esophageal obstruction due to a guar gum preparation (Cal-Bran 3000). *S Afr Med J* 1992; 85: 642–5.

Heaton KW. Concepts of dietary fibre. In: *Dietary Fibre: Chemical and Biological Aspects.* Southgate DAT, Waldron K, Johnson IT, Fenwick GB,. eds. Cambridge: Royal Society of Chemistry, 1990, pp 3–19.

Hellendoorn EW, Noordhoff MG, Slagman J. Enzymatic determination of the indigestible residue (dietary fibre) contents of human food. *J Sci Fd Agric.* 1975; 26: 1461–8.

Henry DA, Mitchell AS, Aylward J, Fung MT, McEwen J, Rohan A. Glucomannan and risk of oesophageal obstruction. *Br Med J* 1986; 292: 591–2.

Hipsley EH. Dietary 'fibre' and pregnancy toxaemia. *Br Med J* 1953; ii: 420–2.

Holland B, Unwin ID, Buss DH. *Cereals and Cereal Products.* Cambridge: Royal Society of Chemistry and MAFF, 1988.

Holland B, Unwin ID, Buss DH. *Vegetables, Herbs and Spices.* Cambridge: Royal Society of Chemistry and MAFF, 1991.

Holland B, Unwin ID, Buss DH. *Fruits and Nuts.* Cambridge: Royal Society of Chemistry and MAFF, 1992.

Holland B, Welch AA, Unwin ID, Buss DH, Paul AA, Southgate DAT. *McCance and Widdowson's The Composition of Foods.* 5th Ed. Cam-bridge: Royal Society of Chemistry, 1991.

Holt S, Heading RC, Cater DC, Prescott LF, Tothill P. Effect of gel-forming fibre on gastric emptying and absorption of glucose and paracetamol. *Lancet* 1979;i: 636–9.

Jacobs LR. Enhancement of rat colon carcinogenesis by wheat bran consumption during the stage of 1,2-dimethylhydrazine administration. *Cancer Res.* 1983; 43: 4057–61.

Jacobs LR. Stimulation of rat colonic crypt cell proliferative activity by wheat bran consumption during the stage of 1,2-dimethylhydrazine administration. *Cancer Res* 1984; 44: 2458–2463

Jacobs LR. Dietary fibre and cancer. *J Nutr* 1987; 117: 1319–21.

Jacobs LR, Lupton JR. Relationship between colonic luminal pH, cell proliferation, and colon carcinogenesis in 1,2-dimethylhydrazine treated rats fed high fiber diets. *Cancer Res* 1986; 46: 1727–34.

Jacobs LR, White FA. Modulation of mucosal cell proliferation in the intestine of rats fed a wheat bran diet. *Am J Clin Nutr.* 1983; 37: 945–53.

James WPT, Branch WJ, Southgate DAT. Calcium binding by dietary fibre. *Lancet* 1978; i: 638–9.

Jenkins AP, Thompson, RPH. Effect of dietary fat on the distribution of mucosal mass and cell proliferation along the small intestine. *Gut* 1992; 33: 224–9.

Jenkins DJA, Wolever TMS, Leeds AR, Gassul MA, Haisman P, Dilawari J, Goff DV, Metz GJ, Alberti KGMM. Dietary fibres, fibre analogues and glucose tolerance: importance of viscosity. *Br Med J* 1978; i: 1392–4.

Jenkins DJA, Wolever TMS, Taylor RH, Barker H, Fielden H, Baldwin JM, Bowling AC, Newman HC, Jenkins AL, Golf DV. Glycaemic index of foods: a physiological basis for carbohydrate exchange. *Am J Clin Nutr.* 1981; 34: 362–6.

Johnson IT, Gee JM. Gastrointestinal adaptation in response to soluble non-available polysaccharides in the rat. *Br J Nutr* 1986; 55: 497–505.

Johnson IT, Gee JM, Mahoney RR. Effect of dietary supplements of guar gum and cellulose on intestinal cell proliferation, enzyme levels and sugar transport in the rat. *Br J Nutr* 1984; 52: 477–87.

Johnson IT, Gee JM, Price K, Curl C, Fenwick GR. Influence of saponins on gut permeability and active nutrient transport *in vitro*. *J Nutr* 1986; 16: 2270–7.

Jung HG, Fahey GC. Nutritional implications of phenolic monomers and lignin: a review. *J Animal Sci* 1983; 57: 206–19.

Kang JY, Dow WF. Unprocessed bran causing intestinal obstruction. *Br Med J* 1979; i: 1249–50.

Koruda MJ, Rolandelli RH, Settle RG, Saul SH, Rombeau JL. The effect of a pectin supplemented elemental diet on intestinal adaptation to massive small bowel resection. *J Parent Ent Nutr* 1986; 10: 343–50.

Livesey G. The energy values of dietary fibre and sugar alcohols for man. *Nutr Res Rev.* 1992; 5: 61–84.

Lund EK, Gee JM, Brown JC, Woods PJ, Johnson IT. Effects of oat gum on the physical properties of the gastrointestinal contents and the uptake of

D-galactose and cholesterol by rat small intestine *in vitro. BR J Nutr.* 1989; 62: 91–101

Lupton JR, Coder DM, Jacobs LR. Influence of luminal pH on rat large bowel epithelial cell cycle. *Am J Physiol* 1985; 249: G382–G388.

McCance RA, Widdowson EM. Mineral metabolism of healthy adults on white and brown bread dietaries. *J Physiol* 1942; 101: 44–85.

McCance RA, Widdowson EM. *The Composition of Foods.* 1st, 2nd and 3rd editions. London: HMSO, 1940, 1946, 1960.

McCance RA, Lawrence RD. The carbohydrate content of foods. Special Report of the Medical Research Council, No. 135. London: HMSO.

McClurken JB, Carp NZ. Bran-induced small intestinal obstruction in a patient with no history of abdominal operation. *Arch Surg* 1988; 123: 98–100.

McIvor AC, Meguid MM, Curtas S, Warren J, Kaplan DS. Intestinal obstruction from gastric bezoar; a complication of fiber containing tube feeds. *Nutr* 1990; 6: 115–7.

Meiser G, Waclawiczek HW, Heinerman M, Boeckl O. Der intermittierende inkomplette Dunndarmileus: Sonographische Diagnostic und Trend beobachtung. *Chirurg* 1990; 6: 651–5.

Merrill AL, Watt BK. Energy value of foods, basis and derivation. US Dept Agric Agriculture Handbook No. 74. Washington, DC: US Government Printing Office, 1990.

Meyer JH, Elashoff YGJ, Reedy T, Fressman J, Amidon G. Effects of viscosity and fluid outflow on postcibal gastric emptying of solids. *Am J Physiol* 1986; 250: G161–G164.

Miller DD, Schricker BR, Rasmussen RR, Van Campen D. An *in vitro* method for estimation of iron availability from meals. *Am J Clin Nutr.* 1981; 34: 2248–56.

Ministry of Agriculture, Fisheries and Food. *Guidelines on Nutritional Labelling.* London: MAFF, 1987.

Ministry of Agriculture, Fisheries and Food. MAFF validated methods for the analysis of foodstuffs. VI Dietary fibre (Colorimetry). *J Assoc Public Anal* 1992; 28: 17–24.

Morse JM, Malloy WX. Esophageal obstruction caused by Cal-Bran. *Gastroenterol* 1990; 98: 805–6.

Morton JF. Tentative correlations of plant usage and esophageal cancer zones. *Econ Bot* 1970; 24: 217–26.

Nachbar MS, Oppenhiem JD. Lectins in the United States diet: a survey of lectins in commonly consumed foods and a review of the literature. *Am J Clin Nutr.* 1980; 33: 2338–45.

Noah ND, Bender AE, Reaidi GB, Gilbert RJ. Food poisoning from raw kidney beans. *Br Med J* 1980; ii: 236–7.

Nyman ME, Björck IM. In vivo effects of phytic acid and polyphenols on the bioavailability of polysaccharides and other nutrients. *J Food Sci* 1989; 54: 1332–5.

Oohashi Y, Kitamura S, Wakabayashi K, Kuwabara N. Irreversibility of degraded carageenan-induced colorectal squamous metaplasia in rats. *Gann* 1979; 70: 391–2.

Opper FH, Isaacs KL, Warshauer DM. Esophageal obstruction with a dietary fiber product designed for weight reduction. *J Clin Gastroenterol* 1990; 12: 667–9.

Painter NS, Burkitt DP. Diverticular disease of the colon; A deficiency disease of Western civilisation. *Br Med J* 1971; ii: 450–4.

Paul AA, Southgate DAT. *McCance and Widdowson's The Composition of Foods.* 4th ed. London: HMSO, 1978.

Pell JD, Gee JM, Wortley GM, Johnson IT. Dietary corn oil and guar gum stimulate intestinal crypt cell proliferation in rats by independent but potentially synergistic mechanisms. *J Nutr* 1992; 122: 2447–56.

Pell J, Johnson IT, Goodlad RA. Fibre, fat and flora. *Gut.* 1993; 34 (Suppl. 4): S59.

Perisse J, Sizaret F, Francois P. The effect of income on the structure of the diet. *Nutrition Newsletter, FAO* 1969; 16:1–9.

Potter JD, McMichael AJ. Diet and cancer of the colon and rectum: a case control study. *J Nat Cancer Inst* 1986; 76: 557–69.

Preston-Martin S, Pike MC, Ross RK, Jones PA, Henderson BE. Increased cell division as a cause of human cancer. *Cancer Res* 1990; 50: 7415–21.

Prosky L, Asp NG, Furda I, Devries JW, Schweizer TF, Harland BF. Vitamins and other nutrients. Determination of total dietary fiber in foods, food products and total diets: interlaboratory study. *J Official Analyt Chem* 1984; 67: 1044–52.

Prosky L, Asp N-G, DeVries JW, Furda I. Determination of insoluble, soluble and total dietary fiber in foods and food products Interlaboratory study. *J Official Analyt Chem* 1988; 71: 1017–23.

Prynne CJ, Southgate DAT. The effects of a supplement of dietary fibre on faecal excretion by human subjects. *Br J Nutr* 1979; 41: 495–503,

Pusztai A, Grant G, de Oliveira JTA. Local (gut) and systemic responses to dietary lectins. *IRCS Med Sci* 1986; 14: 209–10.

Read NW, Welch IMcL, Austen CJ. Swallowing food without chewing: A simple way to reduce postprandial glycaemia. *Br J Nutr* 1986; 5: 43–7.

Ridout CL, Wharf SG, Price KR, Johnson IT; Fenwick GR. UK mean daily intake of saponins - intestine permeabilising factors in legumes. *Food Sci Nutr* 1988; 42F: 111–116.

Ring SG, Gee JM, Whittam M, Orford P, Johnson IT. Resistant starch: Its chemical form in foodstuffs and effect on digestibility *in vitro. Food Chem* 1988; 28: 97–109.

Rosario PG, Gerst PH, Prakash K, Albu E. Dentureless distension: oat bran bezoars cause obstruction. *J Am Geriatric Soc* 1990; 38: 608.

Rossander L, Sandberg A-S, Sandstrom B. The influence of dietary fibre on mineral absorption and utilisation. In: *Dietary Fibre: A Component of Food.* Schweizer TF, Edwards CA, eds. London: Springer Verlag, 1992, pp 197–216.

Rutishauser IHE, Whitehead RG. Energy intake and expenditure in 1–3 year old Ugandan children living in a rural environment. *Br J Nutr* 1972; 28: 145–52.

Sakata T. Stimulatory effect of short-chain fatty acids on epithelial cell proliferation in the rat intestine: a possible explanation for trophic effects of fermentable fibre, gut microbes and luminal trophic factors. *Br J Nutr* 1987; 5: 95–103.

Sakata T, Yajima T. Influence of short chain fatty acids on the epithelial cell division of digestive tract. *Quart J Exp Physiol* 1984; 69: 639–48.

Sandberg A-S, Carlsson N-G, Svanberg U. Effects of inositol tri-, tetra-, penta-, and hexaphosphates on the in vitro estimations of iron availabliity. *J Food Sci* 1989; 54: 159–61.

Saunders RM, Betschart AA. The significance of protein as a component of dietary fiber. *Am J Clin Nutr* 1980; 33: 960–1.

Scheppach W, Burghardt W, Bartram P, Kasper H. Addition of dietary fiber to liquid formula diets: The pros and cons. *J Parent Ent Nutr* 1990; 14: 204–9.

Scheppach W, Sommer H, Kirchner T, Paganelli G, Bartram P, Christl S, Richter F, Dusel G, Kasper H. Effect of butyrate enemas on the colonic mucosa in distal ulcerative colitis. *Gastroenterol.* 1992; 103: 51–6.

Schweizer TF. Dietary fibre analysis. *Lebensmitt Wissen Technol* 1989; 22: 54–9.

Seidner DL, Roberts IM, Smith MS. Esophageal obstruction after ingestion of a fiber-containing diet pill. *Gastroenterol* 1990; 99: 1829–21.

Selvendran RR. The plant cell wall as a source of dietary fibre: chemistry and structure. *Am J Clin Nutr* 1984; 39: 320–7.

Selvendran RR, O'Neill MA. Isolation of cell walls from plant material. In: *Methods of Biochemical Analysis.* Vol. 32. Glick D, ed. New York, John Wiley, 1987, pp 25–145.

Simpson HCR, Simpson RW, Lousley S *et al.* A high-carbohydrate leguminous fibre diet improves all aspects of diabetic control. *Lancet* 1981; i: 1–5.

Slavin JL, Martlett JA. Influence of refined cellulose on human bowel function and calcium and magnesium balance. *Am J Clin Nutr* 1980; 33: 1932–39.

Southgate DAT. Determination of carbohydrates in foods. II Unavailable carbohydrates. *J Sci Food Agric* 1969; 20: 331–336.

Southgate DAT. Non-assimilable components of food. In: *Nutritional Problems in a Changing World.* Hollingsworth DF, ed. London: British Nutrition Foundation, 1973, pp 199–204.

Southgate DAT. Fiber and other unavailable carbohydrates and energy, effects in the diet. In: *Proceedings of Western Hemisphere Nutrition Congress IV.* Acton: American Medical Association Publishing Sciences Group, 1975, pp 51–5.

Southgate DAT. The chemistry of dietary fiber. In: *Fiber in Human Nutrition.* Spiller GA, Amen RJ, eds. New York: Plenum Press, 1976a, pp 31–72.

Southgate DAT. The analysis of dietary fiber. In: *Fiber in Human Nutrition.* Spiller GA, Amen RJ, eds. New York: Plenum Press, 1976b, 73–107.

Southgate DAT. Minerals, trace elements, and potential hazards. *Am J Clin Nutr* 1987; 45: 1256–66.

Southgate DAT. Dietary fibre and the diseases of affluence. In: *A Balanced Diet?* Dobbing J, ed. London: Springer Verlag, 1988, pp 117–39.

Southgate DAT. Conceptual issues concerning the assessment of nutritional bioavailability. In: *Nutrient Bioavailability: Chemical & Biological Aspects.*

Southgate D, Johnson IT, Fenwick GR, eds. Cambridge: Royal Society of Chemistry, 1989, pp 10–12.

Southgate DAT. The dietary fibre hypothesis: A historical perpective. In: *Dietary Fibre: A Component of Food.* Schweizer TF, Edwards CA, eds. London: Springer Verlag, 1992, pp 3–20.

Southgate DAT, Durnin JVGA. Calorie conversion factors: an experimental assessment of the factors used in the calculation of the energy value of human diets. *Br J Nutr* 1970; 24: 517–35.

Standstead H, Klevay LM, Jacob RA *et al..* Effects of dietary fiber and protein level on mineral element metabolism. In: *Dietary Fiber Chemistry and Nutrition.* Inglett GE, Falkenhag SI, eds. New York: Academic Press, 1979, pp 147–156.

Stanten A, Peters HE. Enzymatic dissolution of phytobezoars. *Am J Dig Dis* 1975; 130: 259–61.

Stephen AM, Cummings JH. Mechanism of action of dietary fibre in the colon. *Nature* 1980; 284: 283–4.

Trowell HC. Ischemic heart disease and dietary fiber. *Am J Clin Nutr* 1972; 25: 926–32.

Trowell HC, Southgate DAT, Wolever TMS, Leeds AR, Gassull MA, Jenkins DJA. Dietary fibre redefined. *Lancet* 1976; i: 967.

Truswell AS, Beynen AC. Dietary fibre and plasma lipids: Potential for prevention and treatment of hyperlipidaemia. In: *Dietary Fibre: A Component of Food.* Schweizer TF, Edwards CA, eds. London: Springer Verlag, 1992, pp 295–332.

US Senate Select Committee on Nutrition and Human Needs. *Dietary Goals for the United States.* Washington, DC: US Government Printing Office, 1977.

Van Soest PJ. Use of detergents in the analysis of fibrous feeds. 1 Preparation of fiber residues of low nitrogen content. *J Assoc Official Agric Chem* 1963; 46: 825–9.

Varel VH, Jung HG.Influence of forage phenolics on ruminal fibrolytic bacteria and in vitro fiber degradation. *Appl Env Microbiol* 1986; 52: 275–80.

Wilcox DK, Higgins J, Bertram TA. Colonic epithelial cell proliferation in a rat model of nongenotoxin-induced colonic neoplasia. *Lab Invest* 1992; 67: 405–11.

Wilpart M, Roberfroid M. Intestinal carcinogenesis and dietary fibers: The influence of cellulose or fybogel chronically given after exposure to DMH. *Nutr Canc* 1987; 10: 39–51.

Wolthers MGE. Prediction of the bioavailability of minerals in foods. Thesis, Landbouwuniversitet Wageningen, Neths., 1992.

Wyatt GM, Horn N, Gee JM, Johnson IT. Intestinal microflora and gastrointestinal adaptation in the rat in response to non-digestible dietary polysaccharides. *Br J Nutr* 1988; 60: 197–207.

Index